INTIMATE RELATIONSHIPS IN MEDICAL SCHOOL

To all medical students—
today, yesterday, and tomorrow.

INTIMATE RELATIONSHIPS IN MEDICAL SCHOOL

MICHAEL F. MYERS

SCHOOL

How to Make Them Work

Sage Publications, Inc.
International Educational and Professional Publisher
Thousand Oaks ▪ London ▪ New Delhi

For information:

Sage Publications, Inc.
2455 Teller Road
Thousand Oaks, California 91320
E-mail: order@sagepub.com

Sage Publications Ltd.
6 Bonhill Street
London EC2A 4PU
United Kingdom

Sage Publications India Pvt. Ltd.
M-32 Market
Greater Kailash I
New Delhi 110 048 India

Library of Congress Cataloging-in-Publication Data

Myers, Michael F.
    Intimate relationships in medical school: How to make them work / by Michael F. Myers.
        p. cm. — (Surviving medical school; v. 5)
    Includes bibliographical references (p.) and index.
    ISBN 0-7619-2063-3 (p: acid-free paper)
    1. Physicians—Family relationships. 2. Medical students. 3. Physicians' spouses. I. Title. II. Series.
    R707.2 .M945 2000
    610.69'6—dc21   00-008087

This book is printed on acid-free paper.

00 01 02 03 04 05 06 7 6 5 4 3 2 1

Acquisition Editor:	Rolf Janke
Editorial Assistant:	Heidi Van Middlesworth
Production Editor:	Sanford Robinson
Editorial Assistant:	Victoria Cheng
Copy Editor:	Linda Gray
Typesetter:	Tina Hill
Indexer:	Teri Greenberg
Cover Designer:	Ravi Balasuriya

Contents

Foreword

Many medical students and house staff suffer from stressed-out couple relationships. Receiving little or no help, they tough it out or eventually break up.

Until now, there has been no practical guide, no book specifically designed for medical trainees to strengthen couple relationships and ameliorate disenchantment and disengagement. Using interesting case vignettes and helpful suggestions, Michael Myers, M.D., provides practical information that, if you follow, will strengthen your relationship.

Writing in a reader-friendly style, Dr. Myers assures you that you are not alone in relationship problems, help is readily available, and a hopeful future possible. He conveys the encouraging message that some faculty *do* care about your personal life, not just how well you master pedagogic materials.

Dr. Myers, a psychiatrist with more than 25 years of experience helping medical trainees with relationship issues, is an internationally known clinician and instructor. He and Leah Dickstein, M.D., associate dean of student affairs at the University of Louisville, offer an annual course—Treating Medical Students and Physicians—that sells out each year at the meetings of the American Psychiatric Association.

Clinical professor of psychiatry at the University of British Columbia and director of the Marital Therapy Clinic at St. Paul's Hospital in Vancouver, Dr. Myers is deeply involved in guiding medical trainees and practicing physicians through the vicissitudes of their personal and professional lives. A successful and well-respected author, his book *Doctors' Marriages: A Look at the Problems and Their Solutions* (1988, 1994) targets physicians and their spouses; *How's Your Marriage? A Book for Men and Women* (1998) is geared for the general public. Both have received rave reviews.

Whether or not you're currently involved in an intimate relationship, you will benefit from reading this book and implementing its precepts. Maintaining a viable relationship with an intimate other will be the best buffer you can have against stress and emotional impairment. This book represents the best in primary (i.e., avoiding potential relationship problems) and secondary (i.e., fixing problems before they become deeply entrenched) prevention. I guarantee that you'll learn a lot and will take an important step toward ensuring your present and future well-being.

—Robert Holman Coombs
Professor of Biobehavioral Sciences,
UCLA School of Medicine
Series Editor

Acknowledgments

I wish to thank Plenum Press for permission to adapt material for this book from a chapter on medical student and resident physician marriages in my book *Doctors' Marriages: A Look at the Problems and Their Solutions* (1988, 1994) and American Psychiatric Press, Inc., for permission to adapt from my book *How's Your Marriage? A Book for Men and Women* (1998). I want to thank Dr. Robert Coombs for inviting me to write this book. He has believed in its purpose since the beginning. Thanks as well to the many medical students at UCLA who reviewed the prospectus and supported the need for a book on intimate relationships. I would also like to thank the hundreds of medical students, spouses, partners, and children who have been my patients. You have entrusted me with your care, your very personal struggles, heartaches, and joy. This is your book. Finally, I want to thank my wife Joice, my daughter Briana, and my son Zachary. I could never write a book on intimate relationships without their love. And much more.

Introduction

If you are married or in a committed intimate relationship, you will find this book helpful. I have been listening to the concerns of medical students about their relationships for over 25 years, as a psychiatrist with a subspecialty in physician health, as a director of medical student education, and as a clinical teacher. Although, I myself was not married or in a serious relationship while a medical student, I became both a husband and father during my residency. I haven't forgotten the many stressful days and sleepless nights when things were not going well at home. Nor have I forgotten the agonizing attempts to reconcile my commitment to my patients and studies and my wish to have a life outside of medicine with my wife, children, and friends. I longed for something to read about this dilemma (but there wasn't much back then) or someone to talk to about this. I thought that I was the only one having trouble coping, and I simply felt inadequate and frightened. After my residency and when I began to work in the field, I quickly realized that I was not alone and that many medical students and residents in committed relationships were struggling with the same issues.

By now, you have probably experienced (or have been told that you might experience) some stress simply because you are a medical student. Here are some of the more common sources: adjusting to medical training and deciding that you are in the right field; coping with the volume of material to be learned; grappling with disease and dying patients; confronting ethical dilemmas in health care; balancing academic demands with those of your family; delaying gratification of many of your personal needs; not getting enough time to keep up your interests; for some of you, accepting a decline in academic standing, failing one or more courses, writing supplemental examinations, or repeating a year of medical school; and coping with illness in yourself or a loved one, including family tragedies. All of these can have an impact on intimacy in your life.

This book is for you and your spouse or partner to read. I have tried to discuss the more common sources of conflict in relationships during medical training. I hope that your reading about these matters will give you more information and insight into your struggles and those of your partner. Pay attention to the suggestions that I make about communication, because if you can master some of these techniques and strategies, you will be able to discuss many tough issues much more easily than before. That is key. With good communication skills and an enduring wish to understand and to be close again, you will be proud of your ability to confront and resolve misunderstandings.

I have used lots of case examples throughout this book. They are composites from my practice. I have deliberately disguised details to protect my patients' identities and to preserve their confidentiality and dignity. I hope that you find their stories helpful.

1 We're Not Communicating

Not communicating is one of the most frustrating features of a relationship and comes in many forms. Here are some examples:

- "Our communication with each other is the pits. If I mention anything even slightly critical, Jennifer gets defensive and attacks me."

- "We can talk about school, our families, and our friends. However, if I want to discuss our relationship, Brent shuts down or accuses me of analyzing him."

- "We can't resolve any disagreements. All we do is fight, don't speak for a day or two, then go back to business as usual. The same issue comes up over and over again."

- "We have been together for two years, and yet I don't really know Pete. He won't let me in. I feel so lonely and yet I really love him."

- "Both of us avoid conflict. We both grew up in homes where our parents fought a lot until they divorced. I think we escape into studying and don't let the other know when we feel angry or hurt."

- "I don't feel like having sex anymore. But we never talk. Who feels like making love to a stranger."

- "Claire is like most women; she always wants to talk and gets furious at me because I never have anything to say."

- "Bill is like most men—never wants to talk but always wants sex."

These simple statements embody both quantitative and qualitative complaints of communication troubles. Quantitative equates with "We don't talk enough." Qualitative equates with "We don't communicate with depth, feeling, meaning, vitality, soul." Both can lead to annoyance, exasperation, head-aches, demoralization, sexual avoidance or unresponsiveness, romantic and sexual interest in others, and the end of the relationship.

Quantitative Type

Lots of things can cause quantitative problems with communication. Common in medical student relationships is lack of time. You are both too busy to talk and don't see each other enough to get beyond the basics of "How was your day?" Or you are so preoccupied with classes, clinics, and studying that you don't make the time to relax and talk together. That is, your priority is school, not your relationship. Perhaps you think—erroneously—that relationships will flourish without your attention, time, energy, and love or that your partner will simply understand and be patient, without realizing that that is a lot to ask of someone.

Watch for this warning signal: You don't feel like seeing your partner, or if you are married or are living together, you don't feel like going home at the end of the day. In fact, you find yourself making excuses to stay late, preferring to study in the library, volunteering to take on extra clinical duties, or getting in-volved in more and more extracurricular activities. But you don't have the guts to sit down with your partner and talk about the way that you are feeling. "I don't want to hurt her (him)" is the most common excuse.

Here are two other examples of quantitative problems in communicating:

1. You are spending lots of time together, but the silence is painful. Neither of you seems to have much to say. This may be due to shyness or social awk-wardness, but if you are well into a relationship together and this is a change, then there are probably lots of unspoken matters inhibiting the two of you. Be-ware of the common tendency to avoid being alone together because of this—constantly double-dating, spending time exclusively with your kids, or visiting extended family and friends.

Josh and Sara complained that their lives were so busy that they never got any time alone. I requested that they get out together alone on a date once every two weeks. Several weeks passed and this did-n't happen. They were always too busy with school, committees, friends, and volunteering. I noticed that they never spoke to each other in my waiting room. They said this was because they liked to read my magazines! I also observed that they didn't speak to each other in my office either. They both talked a lot but always to me about the other. I did a role play with each of them to explain what I meant and to emphasize that one-to-one time together is essential in all relationships. Their "date" was very uncomfortable but got easier with practice—along with their taking risks with each other about all the stuff that they had bottled up (Sara's hurt that Josh was not really there for her during a therapeutic abortion; Josh's sense that Sara cared only about her medical school friends and not his dental school friends; Sara's wish to get married soon and Josh's preference to live together for another three to four years).

2. One of you does all the talking and the other listens. Whoever is doing most or all of the talking is probably filling in dead space because the other is silent. A vicious circle gets going: The more the quiet one is quiet, the more the talkative one overtalks.

Caroline and Craig had the same chief complaint—that they were spinning their wheels with each other and wondering if they should get married or not. They had been together for five years but said that they really didn't know each other. What I noticed immediately was their pattern of Caroline's doing all the talking; she started talking immediately and never really paused. I had to keep interrupting. Craig never interrupted her. If I asked a question of the two of them or Craig alone, he would turn to her and she would start—and not stop. I noticed that he appeared to be listening at first but after 30 seconds or so, he'd look around my office, look at my artwork, check out my books, or simply seem a million miles away. Thinking this might be all due to anxiety at meeting together with a psychiatrist, I asked about it, but they said that this was their pattern everywhere whether home alone or with friends and family. I suggested to Caroline that she stop at the end of statements or questions to Craig and not say anything until he responded. I suggested to Craig that he speak first more often and that he try to reveal more about himself to Caroline—that is, that self-disclosure leads to intimacy.

Qualitative Type

There are several kinds of qualitative problems when communicating or trying to communicate.

- The amount of talk may be fine, but it is very superficial, inane, boring, or self-centered.
- The language that you use may be sterile, cold, pedantic, distant, intellectualized, and devoid of feeling. Your medical terminology may spill into your personal life: An overstated example might be, "Would you like to have coitus?" instead of "Let's make love."
- Your language and speech may be provocative, hostile, and sarcastic: "I didn't know you were a genius—and you're so modest about it!"
- Perhaps your words are threatening: "If you don't come with me to the doctor, I'm leaving you!"
- Perhaps your words are mean: "Keep eating that ice cream and Weight Watchers will be recruiting you for their next year's poster child."
- Maybe you resort to name-calling: "You controlling bitch!" or "What a selfish bastard you are!"
- Maybe you resort to swearing: "F__ you!"
- Maybe you engage in exhausting talk that goes nowhere: That is, you go round in circles with each other. And if this occurs at bedtime, you may be up late and have trouble falling off to sleep.

The Consequences of Poor Communication

- Demoralization
- Fatigue
- A sense of hopelessness and loss of faith in the relationship
- Depression
- Drinking and other drug use (e.g., smoking marijuana)
- Physical symptoms (e.g., headaches, backaches, gastrointestinal upsets, recurrent outbreaks of genital herpes)
- Distancing from each other
- Sexual withdrawal, loss of sexual satisfaction
- Extramarital relationships

What to Do

- Don't despair: Communication problems are ubiquitous and common to all re-lationships in varying degrees. Look on your recognition of communication impasses as a wakeup call, a challenge, a signal that the two of you care about each other.

- Remember that how you communicate with others—your friends, classmates, professors, patients, and family members—is very different from and easier than communicating with your partner. Being engaged in an intimate relationship means that you can easily feel exposed, hurt, enraged, jealous, put down, shamed, and defensive. And this is why communication can go haywire!

- Also remember that easy communication does not equate with intelligence. Therefore, do not assume that you are immune or that you can figure it all out logically. One of the most common statements is this: "I'm very frustrated. I'm not dumb for godsakes; I'm a medical student. But my wife and I can't discuss the weather without fighting!"

- Make your relationship communication a high priority in your life. Don't avoid dealing with it. Don't throw yourself into your studies to the exclusion of talking at home. It's risky not to heed your partner's wishes to talk. And it can get dangerous. Some relationship violence is rooted in a partner's stubborn refusal to talk and to listen.

- No one is born with an innate ability to communicate in intimate relationships. And not uncommonly, many medical students do not believe that their parents were the best role models in how to talk in marriage.

- All human beings are influenced by their families of origin, their genetic endowment, their exposure to other couples and families, and their own capacity to learn from what worked and did not work in their own previous relationships and marriages. Think about some of the many factors that have shaped you and account for who you are today.

- Take risks with each other. Be honest and open with your feelings. There are ways to talk about difficult subjects with grace and mutual respect.

- Be prepared for defensiveness in yourself and your partner, for hurt and angry feelings, and for counterattacks. Name these phenomena and talk about them with each other.

- Set aside time to communicate—daily, weekly, biweekly. Be creative in the many ways that you can communicate with each other—face-to-face, telephone, "Post-it" notes, cards, thoughtful gestures, e-mail, and gifts.

- Which setting(s) work for the two of you? At home? Where in the home? Away from home? In a restaurant? Coffee shop? At the park? In a car? Opposite each other or beside each other? Sitting or in motion (e.g., walking, riding bicycles).

- Preface comments that may hurt with a positive statement: For example, "Randy, we gotta talk. First of all, I love you to bits. You're the best thing that's ever happened to me, but we need to talk about your dope smoking. It's really beginning to bug me. You're smoking daily now, and I think you're getting addicted."

- Apologize when it's appropriate: "I'm sorry I was so mean to you last night. I think that I was more wiped out from being on call and up all night than I realized. I feel so much better today now that I'm rested."

- When you don't feel an apology is warranted, try something like this: "Can we talk about last night? What happened? Suddenly I felt that you were attacking me, and I hadn't done anything wrong. And then I found myself coming at you with both barrels. What're your thoughts about last night?"

- Report your feelings: Don't start an analytical dissection of your partner and your relationship with him or her.

- No name-calling: Apologize when you catch yourself or when you're reminded that you have done it again.

- Avoid absolutes: "You never clean the sink after you shave." "You always look at me with disgust when I make a mistake in my grammar."

- Put your complaints in the form of a request: Instead of saying, "You're so selfish and couldn't care less about me and my feelings," say, "Would you please call me from the hospital and let me know if you're going to be late? That way I can more easily plan my evening. Thanks."

- Interrupt: There are occasions when you should signal if your partner is going from subject to subject and you want to respond to matters one at a time. If you don't signal or if your partner refuses to stop, you will become annoyed and begin to tune out.

- Don't interrupt: There are occasions when it is rude to interrupt. Especially if your intent is not to respond or make a relevant point but to change the subject or to control the conversation or to bully your partner.

- Don't hold grudges: It's OK to sulk when you are angry, but 24 hours is plenty. When people sulk for more than a day, they have usually become self-righteous, self-indulgent, and punitive—not a very mature way to function in an intimate relationship.

2 Is Communicating Supposed to Be This Hard?

The answer to the question is a resounding "Yes" and a resounding "No." There are times in all relationships when communication is, or feels, completely impossible, only to be followed by tremendous facility in communication in the same relationship at another time. The bottom line, however, is that no human being is born with innate wisdom in communicating easily at all times and with all people.

It is known that when individuals grow up in a family where open and direct communication among family members is not only common but also honored, the offspring learn to talk with others outside the family much more easily. In other words, this is a family in which individuals are encouraged to be straightforward and as clear as possible regarding their feelings and thoughts on matters relevant to family life. This tends to be an ideal, however; very few families in North America are structured in this way.

If you would like to have the best communication possible in your intimate relationship, there are at least four attitudes that you must possess or strive for:

1. You must desire and be willing to communicate directly and clearly at all times.

2. You must be prepared to take risks.

3. You must be prepared to reveal painful or embarrassing things about yourself from time to time.

4. You must be prepared to hear upsetting things said to you by your spouse or partner.

7

Medical students vary tremendously in their ability to know and identify what their needs are and in their willingness to communicate clearly when involved in an intimate relationship with someone else. Some years ago, Dr. Clifford Sager (1976, pp. 19-20), a psychiatrist and marital therapist, suggested three different levels of communication in intimate relationships: conscious and verbalized, conscious but not verbalized, and beyond awareness.

Conscious and Verbalized

You are using this level of communication when you are talking about matters that you are aware of and have absolutely no difficulty expressing to your partner or spouse. This type of communication is generally pleasant, flows freely, and, usually, goal oriented. It is easy to solve problems with this level of communication. Most individuals feel listened to, and there is a sense of being understood. This is the clearest and most direct form of communication. When the majority of communication is like this, couples bask in a sense of comfort, achievement, function (as opposed to dysfunction), and solidarity with each other.

Conscious but Not Verbalized

This type of communication is more complicated than the above. In this form of communication, you are aware of certain thoughts and feelings that you don't express. Why not? There are lots of reasons.

- Perhaps you have never been very open or communicative with anyone.
- You may be a quiet, shy, or private person.
- Perhaps you were raised in a home where the atmosphere was not very expressive; no one really talked much about anything.
- Perhaps you were raised in a home where you were put down, reprimanded, or physically beaten for expressing your true feelings or opinions.
- You may be monitoring or censoring what you say because you learned very early in this relationship that some subjects are taboo or that some subjects precipitate very strong emotions. For example, you have made your partner or spouse cry, you have hurt him, you have made her feel sad, you have made him very angry, you have made her feel guilty, or you have made him feel anxious.
- You may also shut down thoughts and feelings because you learned earlier in this relationship that if you disclosed them, this led to frightening behavior in your

partner. Examples include your partner's yelling at you, hitting you, forcing sex on you, getting drunk, sulking, or walking out on you.

For all of the reasons above and perhaps more, at this level of communication, many issues never get talked about. Therefore, the talk and interaction between couples stays at a very superficial, polite, or mundane level.

Beyond Awareness

This level of communication is even more complicated. It is impossible for you to discuss those conflicts because you are not even aware of them. Why? Because the conflicts are unconscious. How do you access them? You may get glimpses of them or fragments of them from dreams you recall on awakening. If you pay attention to the themes or mood of your dreams, including your day-dreams, you may get some insight into the unexpressed conflicts you are avoiding. For example, if you have a repetitive dream of being the victim of aggression, this may indicate a problem in your relationship. Or if you are the perpetrator of aggression in a dream, that may also be a clue to how you are dominating your partner. Other types of themes in dreams can be revealing: being lost, running away, feeling trapped, and being sexually or emotionally involved with someone other than your partner or spouse. You may also get other insights into your unconscious and the unexpressed feelings and ideas there by paying attention to what you talk about (or have been told that you talk about) when you are disinhibited from alcohol. Partners and spouses are sometimes quite surprised, even shocked, at the things said by a loved one when he or she has been drinking. These feelings do not tend to be expressed when the individual is sober. Sarcasm is also another clue. If you find yourself speaking sarcastically or perceive sarcasm in your partner, this often indicates unconscious hostility toward the other. You may not be aware of this in yourself until or if it is pointed out to you by your partner or spouse or by a close friend.

Here is an example that illustrates some of the matters that I have mentioned above:

Alison and Tim were both medical students. Alison was in third-year medicine and Tim was in fourth year. They had been dating for two years and began living together six months before coming to see me. They were engaged and hoped to be married in about a year, but they had some concerns about their communication with each other as well as about their sexual relationship.

Both Alison and Tim felt that they had a lot in common. Because they were both medical students, they could easily talk about their field of study. They were also both competitive athletes and enjoyed working out together and had many friends, both in their class and outside their class, who were like-minded. They each came from families in which one or both parents were physicians. What was troubling for each of them, though, was that they were not able to talk about difficult subjects without the other one getting "super upset." They especially could not talk easily about their sexual relationship for two reasons: Tim found the subject rather embarrassing to talk about, and Alison tended to feel blamed whenever the subject came up.

My individual visits with each of them were illuminating. Tim came from a family in which there was never really any arguing or fighting to any degree. He remembered one occasion when his father yelled at his mother: She broke into tears and ran to the bedroom, his father sat at the dinner table feeling guilty, and that was the end of that. He said that everybody was always "nice" to each other. He described their home also as very conservative, and there was certainly never any discussion about sexual matters, not even in the abstract. His father worked very long hours as a cardiologist, and his mother was an "undiagnosed and untreated" alcoholic. She had trained as a nurse but never returned to paid work outside the home once she began to have a family.

Alison's family was different. Her parents were both physicians and on the "fast track." Both of them worked very long hours and rarely saw each other. She and her two brothers were raised by a succession of nannies. Her mom and dad were frequently out of town at medical meetings but were rarely away together. She described her parents as having "a professional marriage." She went on to say, "Their number one priority is medicine, number two is us, and each other about six." One of the most significant events, and the most traumatic, in Alison's upbringing was that she was date-raped at her high school grad. She had not told anyone about this except a close girlfriend. Since that awful night, though, she had always felt sexually nervous about men.

In the visits that I had with Alison and Tim together, I emphasized how important it was for each of them to begin to talk with each other about their families and how they grew up. They had not really done this in any detailed way. This was a very helpful exercise and experience for the two of them because they came to know each other much more intimately. They also found themselves remembering difficult times in their backgrounds that they had never shared with each other.

To tackle the sexual difficulty that they had with each other, I recommended to Alison in an individual visit that she give some thought to telling Tim about being raped when she graduated from high school. She did this, and Tim was very understanding and compassionate in his response to her. He had lots of questions for her, and this helped her to talk about the more difficult parts. The details, in turn, helped Tim become more comfortable in discussing sexual matters and ways in which people can dominate and control each other in relationships.

Things went very smoothly for several weeks, and the two of them felt much more committed to each other than they had ever felt. They earnestly planned their wedding. However, about three months before the wedding, they had a major crisis. Tim had gotten very drunk at a party and came home very late at night. Not only was he rough with her in pushing to make love, but he was also sarcastic and angry. He made some reference to the subject of rape. Fortunately, Alison got him to stop, and he passed out on the couch. The next day, he felt terrible and very remorseful about his behavior. The two of them went out for a walk together, and with a great deal of hesitancy and shame, Tim told Alison that he had "almost raped" a girlfriend in high school after getting stoned on marijuana. He had never talked about this before with anyone. Talking about it was a great release for him. He cried a lot and expressed a lot of guilty feelings about his forceful and immature behavior.

The above example illustrates elements of Dr. Sager's three levels of communication: Consciousness and verbalized, conscious but not verbalized, and beyond awareness. You can see how much communication at the first level,

although polite and smooth, is not really adequate for high-functioning couples. Communicating at a conscious but previously nonverbalized level (i.e.,
Alison's having been raped) led to a sense of relief in Alison and Tim as well as
a greater sense of solidarity and enhanced intimacy. They were also better able
to resolve problems. And finally, communication at a previously unconscious
level led to even more understanding and mutual sensitivity because of the very
painful and shameful experience from Tim's past.

What Were You Taught About Communication While You Were Growing Up?

It will help you to have a better understanding of any difficulties you are having
in your relationship or marriage if you give some thought to the marriage or
marriages of your parents. Whether you like it or not, your parents were the
first, if not the only, role models you were exposed to in terms of how two
adults communicate with each other in a committed relationship. However,
given the high rates of divorce and remarriage in North America over the past
couple of decades, many of you are "adult children of divorce." In fact, some of
you may have lived through more than one divorce of your parents.

Let me list a few of the many possibilities that characterize the growing-up
years of today's medical students:

- You were raised by two parents who had a reasonably happy marriage that continues until this day.

- Your parents divorced when you were eight years old, and your father remarried
  within two years. Your mother never remarried, and you worry about her; she
  seems lonely or she seems bitter.

- Perhaps you were raised by a single mother who was never married; you have no
  knowledge of your father whatsoever.

- Your parents divorced when you were six years old, and your father remarried and
  divorced twice more; your mother remarried only once, but she is in a miserable
  and very unhappy second marriage.

- Your mother died when you were eleven years old, and your father never dated
  again or remarried.

- You grew up in a series of foster homes, never living in one of them for more than
  two years.

- Your mother is lesbian and has been in a stable relationship for many years; you
  were conceived by donor insemination.

- Your parents divorced when you were three years old, and you have no memory of their ever being together; you have grown up in a joint custody arrangement, spending one week at Mom's house and one week at Dad's house until you became a young adult.

- You were raised in a home that was intact, but you never saw your father because his work took him out of town continually.

- You do not really know your parents as role models or how to communicate because you were sent off to boarding school when you were 10 years old.

- You have never really thought of your parents' form of communication with each other because they have always been in survivor mode; they were refugees to this country, arrived penniless, and have worked night and day to build a life here and send their children to college.

Don't forget that how we communicate in our intimate relationships is more than a by-product of what we learned or didn't learn from our parents' form of communication with each other. We are also genetically influenced. For example, if my father is or was an alcoholic and communicated in a particular way under the influence of alcohol, I may vow never to speak like that to my spouse or children. However, I may be at risk for developing alcoholism and will need to appreciate my vulnerability and need to treat alcohol with absolute respect—or not drink at all. If my mother was prone to recurrent depression and when she was ill she retreated to her room for days on end and did not speak, I may tend to shut down verbally also, not just because of what I learned from her but because I am vulnerable to clinical depression myself.

You might find it helpful to think about the following questions:

- In what ways is my intimate relationship or marriage similar to or different from the marriage or marriages of my parents?

- How am I like my mother in how I talk and communicate with others, and how am I like my father?

- When my parents speak to each other, do they express feelings much?

- Do my parents differ in how much they express emotion?

- When I was growing up, how affectionate were my parents with each other? Did they have nicknames for each other and call each other "honey" or "dear"? Was there much open affection between the two of them—hugs, kisses, holding hands, and so on?

- What were my parents' arguments or fights like? Constructive? Destructive?

- How did my parents deal with stress? Negotiation? Compromise? Drinking? Overspending? Overeating?

If you spend time on these questions and share your answers with each other, you will have much more insight into yourself as well as into your partner. This knowledge will help you to change and to forge bonds with each other. These questions are part of the developmental given that all of us are shaped by a blend of biological, psychological, social, cultural, political, and economic factors. All of these forces contribute to the needs, values, attitudes, and expectations that we bring into our intimate relationships and marriages. As you can see, these questions, and any others that you may think are relevant, are directed at you and not your partner. This is very important, because until you are ready to ask yourself these questions with courage and honesty, it is very difficult if not impossible for you to communicate constructively and with maturity in your chosen relationship.

Do Men and Women Communicate Differently in Their Intimate Relationships?

The answer is, Yes. In general, men tend not to be aware of their feelings quite as much as women do. They may therefore appear to be cooler, more private, more self-contained, and less reactive. That is not to say that their feelings are not somewhere inside. This is the reason that many women in marriage describe feeling lonely. Their common complaint is that their husbands or boyfriends don't talk to them enough or that they do not share inner and personal thoughts and emotions. Many women state that they do a lot of "reading between the lines" or "second-guessing" with their men. This difference between women and men is probably constitutional. It just is that way. This does not mean that one gender is better than the other, or communicates better than the other, or that one is normal and the other is not. Just different.

It is important for women to know that men who don't talk much may still be communicating a great deal to them. Their silence may be a form of passive-aggressive communication. Their being absent from them or withdrawn may say a lot about their mood. When they pour themselves into study or work, that might mean a lot. Men also communicate a lot when they hold back their feelings, when they drink too much, when they make persistent and unwelcome sexual demands, and when they become aggressive, threatening, or violent. These are all forms of communication, but they are oblique, confusing, inappropriate, and unhealthy. Men need to understand that there is a powerhouse of control in these actions and that when they behave like this, they are usually destroying their wives' self-esteem and self-worth and making their wives feel unsafe and certainly not secure or close in their marriages.

Here are two examples of difficulties in communication:

Brenda was a first-year medical student, and her husband Doug was an accountant. Brenda began the visit by stating that they had a serious problem in communication. When I asked her what she meant by this, she went on to say that Doug was a workaholic. She complained that he worked seven days a week and that she rarely saw him except for a few hours in the evenings. When he was home, she found him tired and not very communicative. More specifically, he did not really describe much about his day nor did he seem to show any interest in Brenda's day at school. She stated, "The only time he is tender to me is when he wants to make love. Sometimes this is 45 minutes after he has arrived home, and we haven't exchanged 10 words the whole day. I certainly don't find this a turn-on, and lately I feel nothing but turned off." Doug then spoke: "She's right about our sex life. Lately it's just awful. I don't understand Brenda. You'd think after being in classes all day and studying all evening that she would look forward to a little fun. Accounting is kind of boring; I don't expect Brenda to be interested in it."

As the visit went on, I found Brenda and Doug to be quite wound up. They both seemed to have a lot to say, and they kept interrupting each other and disagreeing with virtually everything that the other person said. Neither seemed to be listening to what the other was saying. At one point in the interview when Brenda was giving a detailed description of the barrenness of their life together, Doug reached for a book off my bookshelf, opened it up, and started reading it. Brenda didn't miss a beat. I cut in to ask her if she noticed what just happened. She responded with, "Of course I did. I don't pay any attention anymore to Doug's rudeness. He's the same way when we make love. We have a TV in the bedroom, and I think he is more interested in CNN than in my pleasure."

At the end of the visit, my sense was that these two individuals did indeed still love each other, but they were both very unhappy and demoralized. They also felt very misunderstood by each other, and both were uncertain as to whether marital therapy could help.

I made the following suggestions to Doug and Brenda:

- Try to listen to each other and do not interrupt.
- Do not speak any longer than one minute, and give your partner an opportunity to respond.
- You will have to accept that you have a lot of unhappy history with each other and that you must begin with a new attitude and a clean slate.
- You have made the decision to go to a trained professional for help. Try to remain hopeful about the process.
- By all means get the TV out of the bedroom!

* * *

Kathy was an occupational therapist working in a neurological rehab center, and her husband Ben was a final-year medical student. When I asked the two of them why they had come to see me, Ben started first. "We have an excellent marriage except that Kathy is hypersensitive." With that, Kathy started to laugh hilariously and could not stop. Soon she had Ben laughing. She then went on to say, "You took the words right out of my mouth. I also think that we have an excellent marriage except that *you* are hypersensitive." When I asked each of them to give examples of what they meant by hypersensitive, they began to tell anecdotes in which they tried to give feedback to the other that resulted in defensiveness. What I noticed, however, was how crudely they spoke to each other and how much they used inflammatory and provocative language.

Here is one of the examples that Ben used to illustrate Kathy's defensiveness. "Last week was my birthday. After we each had a huge slice of chocolate cake and ice cream, Kathy said that she was going to have seconds. I told her that she had better not, that she was getting pretty fat and I didn't want her to end up looking like her mother who I think has really let herself go. Well, my little suggestion propelled Kathy into orbit. She went on to call me every name in the book, told me that I always picked on her, that I never said anything complimentary ever, and that I was beginning to get a bit of a pot belly myself."

Here is one of the examples that Kathy used to illustrate Ben's hyper-sensitivity: "I told Ben that I thought that he needed to study harder. I thought I was being gentle and supportive. When I told him that my father, who is an endocrinologist on faculty here at the medical school, agreed with me, Ben turned on me. He told me that I was *just* an occupational therapist and didn't know anything about medical students. He went on to say that he thought my father was one of the worst endocrinologists in the city, and he wouldn't send his diabetic dog to him. Needless to say, I slept on the couch that night."

I made the following suggestions to Ben and Kathy:

- Watch your choice of words and the tone of your "constructive criticism."
- Refrain from using the terms *always, never,* and *just.*
- Do not compare each other with family members.
- Be more alert to a better time to bring up delicate issues.
- Accept that it is normal to have a knee-jerk reaction of defensiveness when you feel criticized. It is part of feeling hurt and vulnerable. Simply acknowledge it and carry on talking.

These two vignettes illustrate a few of the more common types of communication problems in couples. When communication breaks down, it is a twofold process. This process includes both the "what" and the "how." What we communicate is the content, and how we communicate is the process. These two are closely connected. In other words, what we talk about in our relationships dictates how we communicate. The more painful or upsetting the subject is for you or your partner, the more difficult it is to talk about. Hence, your communication patterns with each other can become blocked or very confusing.

Reference

Sager, C. J. (1976). *Marriage contracts and couple therapy.* New York: Brunner/Mazel.

3 Listening[1]

We always tend to think that we listen well when we are communicating with our spouses or partners. However, listening is easier said than done. It is a very active process that requires a lot of attention. Hence, it is no surprise that our listening can be handicapped if we have a lot on our minds, we are preoccupied, too many people are talking at once, the TV is on, we're in the middle of reading a book, or someone comes to the front door.

Listening is the bedrock of good communication. Here are some factors that commonly contribute to a breakdown in listening and some processes that may get in the way when you are listening to your spouse or partner and what he or she is saying to you.

Comparing

If you are busy comparing what your spouse is saying to you with someone else, then you will not be able to listen with attention. Here are some examples of comparing: She says, "Don't you think you've had enough to drink?" He replies, "Don't you think you've had enough potato chips?" Or she says, "I wish you were home more." He says, "I'm home a lot more than Stan, and he's a medical student too." Or he says, "What have you been doing all day? The bathroom looks like a cyclone hit it." She says, "What have you been doing all day? The kitchen floor hasn't been mopped in a month."

Mind Reading

In this situation, you are so busy anticipating what your spouse is thinking or going to say that you really don't listen to what he or she does say: He says, "I know you're angry with me for being late again, but I couldn't help it. The lab

18

ran late, and I missed my bus coming home." She says, "What I was about to say was do you want spaghetti and meatballs or hamburgers for dinner?"

Rehearsing

In this situation, you are feeling tense, attacked, or put down. You are feeling defensive and your partner continues to talk to you. You are not able to pay attention to him or her because you are so angry and feeling so criticized that you are preparing your response, which is probably a counterattack: She says, "I should have paid more attention to your mother. She told me that you were a little boy and that she waited on you hand and foot. By the way, Carol called today and she and Brandon want us to come over on Saturday night to their home. It's their third anniversary and they are having a barbecue. Do you want to go?" He says, "I should have listened to your father when I picked you up on our first date. He told me that you were a princess and that you like everything your own way."

Filtering

In this situation, you pick up only on certain things that are said to you or about you. Therefore, a lot of the dialogue is missed: She says, "How was my day? I've had a great day. I had two responses to my job application. Both of them are first-rate dental offices. I've got interviews set up this Thursday and this Friday. I ran into Hal at the gym. He told me that the pathology exam was unreal. Cycling back I had a flat tire, but I was able to fix it myself with the new kit that we bought last summer on our cycling trip. But I didn't bring sunscreen with me, and now I've got a heck of a sunburn. Do you think that we should hang the Modigliani print here in the kitchen or in the hallway?" He says, "I think I've failed the pathology exam."

Judging

In this situation, you are listening to your partner or spouse talk about or describe a situation, and you either interrupt or respond with words that rankle. It is not what your partner expected; he or she might shut down, and you are left wondering what went wrong: He says, "How was my day? Pretty good overall for the first day of classes. With the usual orientation pep talks, and they let us off early so that we could take care of banking and stuff like our student loans. There's a new woman in our class who was in second year last year but failed. I went over to her and welcomed her to the class and introduced her to some of the others in our class. She seems like a really neat woman. She developed some kind of an illness last year that caused her to miss a lot of school, and that's why she's doing second year all over again." She says, "She probably had a breakdown. Why else would she be so evasive about an illness?" He says, "Why do you always jump to conclusions about people that you don't even know?" She says, "Stop getting so defensive. You wouldn't even have intro- duced yourself to a new student in the class if the student was a guy."

Dreaming

In this situation, you have trouble listening and concentrating because you are preoccupied. You are off in fantasyland or daydreaming: She says, "Martha called today. She had the baby. Can you imagine $10\frac{1}{2}$ pounds, and she pushed it out without a tear. No forceps. No cesarean section. They are going to call him Bentley. I don't really like the name; it's too androgynous. What do you think?" He says "Who called today?"

Identifying

When you identify with what your spouse is saying, you may feel fine with what you have done. By recording a similar or identical experience to your spouse, you feel good that you have something in common and can share what those experiences are. However, identifying with your partner's experience takes away from the uniqueness of that experience for your partner. He or she may also feel dismissed because you do not ask any questions or ask him or her to explain the experience in more detail: She says, "You'll never guess what happened to me today? Dr. Burman came up to me after rounds and asked me if I'd made a decision yet about a summer research project. When I told him no, he asked me to consider his division. He was familiar with my undergraduate work in immunology, and he wants me to consider coming aboard his research on thyroid antibodies. Can you believe it? I've never been so excited in my life." He says, "When I was in medical school, I had so many profs approaching me about their summer research projects that I rejected them all. I'm glad that I went traveling to Afghanistan. I think I learned more there than I ever would stuck here for the summer."

Advising

This is a not uncommon gender problem. It is much more common for men to advise their partners or wives than the other way around: She says, "I had another tense moment with my lab partner today in anatomy. I don't know what it is. She just doesn't seem to like me. I spoke to Rochelle about it. She's great. I always feel so good after talking with her. Anatomy is so hard and involves so much memorization that I think our entire group is feeling nervous about the test coming up next week. I think that I'll probably . . ." He says, "I think you should ask to be transferred. You go on and on about her every other day." She says, "I didn't ask for advice." He says "Then why do you keep bringing her up? She says, "Because it helps me to get it off my chest." He says, "Oh."

Sparring

If you and your partner are sparring with each other, you will know what that feels like. It is usually representative of some type of underlying relationship tension that is not being directly talked about. It could be that the two of you do not trust each other very well or you are engaged in some kind of power struggle. You find yourselves arguing a lot, putting down what the other is saying, nit-picking over little things, and having major debates about very simple matters.

Being Right

If you have been accused of behaving like you were always right in an argument or discussion, then you should take a look at that. No one is ever always right. You may not be aware of how arrogant you sound or seem to be if you are never wrong. If you have a pathological need to be right at all times, this may be a defense against some anxiety within you or embarrassment if you are occasionally wrong. Although that is human, you may have difficulty accepting that in yourself. People who are "always right" tend to be very competitive or have problems with their self-esteem: She says (looking toward the barbecue), "The hot dogs smell great. I'm starving. Where's the mustard?" He says, "Don't tell me you forgot it." She says, "Well, you're the one who packed all the food." He says, "No, you packed the potato chips." She says, "But I heard you ask in the kitchen, 'Where's the mustard?' and I told you." He says, "No, I didn't say that at all." She says, "Steve, just admit it; you forgot the mustard."

He says, "No, I did not forget the mustard. You forgot the mustard." She says, sarcastically, "Sorry, I forgot, you're always right. It must have been me who once again screwed up."

Derailing

If you derail a conversation that you are having with your spouse, you suddenly change the subject. In other words, you stop listening because you don't find what he or she is saying is very interesting, you feel bored, or you are so preoccupied with your own stuff that you are not very generous in listening to the statements of your partner or spouse. But people also can derail a conversation if the content of what their spouse is saying is upsetting them. In other words, if you feel nervous, ashamed, guilty or angry, you might change the subject so that you don't have to feel those unpleasant emotions: He says, "I made a diagnostic coup today, Honey. This 21-year-old woman came into the emergency room with pain in the right lower quadrant. It was crampy and had been going on for about four hours. She was also pretty nauseated and had been vomiting most of the night. She also had this very intriguing rash all over the lower part of her body. She was an intravenous drug user. When I began to examine her in front of Dr. Campbell, my attending physician . . ." She says, interrupting, "Oh I keep forgetting to tell you, your brother Peter called again. He wants to know whether or not you're going to bring your kayak with you on the trip or whether you're going to use his old one. The one he had before he got his new one."

In this example, it's hard to know whether or not the woman was bored with her husband's clinical stories, especially if this is a pattern that she is finding annoying—and egocentric. Or is she "raining on his parade" when he's trying to share his excitement about his diagnostic coup?

Placating

If you are placating your partner or spouse, you are not really giving him or her your complete and undivided attention. You may be responding in a verbal or nonverbal way that is somewhat insincere and that is also shutting him or her down prematurely: She says, "I'm really struggling on this new rotation. I know for sure that I will never be able to be a pediatric oncologist. Dying kids are too hard on me emotionally. It just isn't fair. I'm looking after a six-year-old right now with an inoperable brain tumor, and even with chemotherapy, his prognosis is grim. He'll be dead within three months." He says, "Sad work. Maybe you should do radiology. Let's go to the gym."

How Can I Listen More Effectively?

Here are four suggestions that you might find helpful:

1. *Listen actively.* Pay close attention to what your spouse or partner has just said. Try paraphrasing what you think he or she has said: "Let me see if I understand what you have just said. Are you saying that Cecilia broke up with Mark or Mark broke up with Cecilia?" Another way of listening actively is to ask questions about what your partner has just said. For example, "Do you mean that you feel kind of upset—upset-sad, upset-angry, upset-hurt?" Another form of active listening is to give your partner some feedback after you have listened to what he or she has said: "You seem kind of hurt. Do you think that you were expecting a promotion too?"

2. *Listen with empathy.* Try to put yourself in your spouse's position, and try to get a sense of what he or she is feeling. Make statements such as, "How frustrating!" "You must be really furious?" "Oh, my God! I can't believe it."

3. *Listen with openness.* If you and your spouse or partner have been together for a while, there is a tendency for communication to become short-circuited. You jump to conclusions about what your partner is going to say or what he or she might be feeling. It is extremely important not to respond in a habitual and rote way. Be patient. Wait until your partner has finished. Don't judge. If you are used to finishing people's sentences and responding before they are finished, this will be hard for you.

4. *Listen with awareness.* If you are having trouble concentrating on what your spouse is saying, ask him or her to stop for a moment; explain that you are having trouble paying attention. You may need to go with him or her to another room. Make sure you turn off the TV. If you are driving in busy traffic and your partner is talking, ask him or her to wait until the traffic is less congested or until you reach your destination. Turn down the radio if the volume is too high. If you think your spouse is speaking too quickly, ask him or her to slow down. If you are simply tired or preoccupied or not feeling well, by all means let your partner or spouse know that, rather than pretending that you are listening.

What Are Some Ways in Which We Can Communicate Better With Each Other?

Here are some suggestions that work for a lot of people. This list is not meant to be inclusive. Some of these suggestions may not interest you, whereas some of the others will have more appeal.

1. If you need to bring up a difficult or sensitive subject, prepare or rehearse what you are going to say and how you are going to say it. Even make a few notes if you think that will be helpful. If you feel that you would like your partner to read what you have written first and then the two of you can discuss it, by all means do that. In fact, letter writing can be a very effective way of communicating when you feel that your spouse or partner just does not get it.

2. Be sure that your spouse is in the mood to talk to you. If he or she is not in the mood right at that moment, then let your partner know that there is something you would like to speak with him or her about later. And if it is quite serious and on your mind, let that be known as well.

3. Use active listening as described above.

4. Try to be as positive as possible. Try to put your complaint about your partner into the form of a request: "When you do the laundry, please wash the whites separate from the coloreds." This will be much more effective than a criticism such as, "Whoever taught you to do laundry? You've mixed all of the whites with the coloreds. You've ruined my new T-shirt from the Gap."

5. Use "I" messages: Instead of, "You really embarrassed me at the party last night. I think you had too much to drink and you were crawling all over Dan." Try, "I'd like to talk about what happened last night at the party, because I'm feeling quite upset."

6. Avoid "you" messages: Instead of, "You never tell me you love me anymore." Try, "I really need to hear you tell me that you love me. As the years go on, I feel more and more insecure."

7. Be specific. Don't bring up events or upsets that happened a year ago; stick to the most recent problem. Don't make sweeping generalizations based on the most recent example: Instead of, "Can we talk about the expenses on the MasterCard for this month. And last month. And the month before and the month before that. In fact, I think you have a spending compulsion, and I'd like to talk about that." Try, "Could we talk about the expenses on the MasterCard for this month?"

8. Stay focused. Once again don't bring up a list of past examples of fights and shortcomings. Don't compare your spouse with his or her least favorite relative. Don't give an example of someone you think does a much better job than

your spouse does: "Your cooking really is pathetic. My mother was a lousy cook too. My last girlfriend was a bitch, but boy, she could cook. It's only August and I'm already dreading Christmas dinner."

9. Try an experiment whereby each of you work at changing some behavior over the next week or two. It is essential that both of you are working on something simultaneously. If you are trying to break a long-standing habit, be aware that you may slip and do it automatically. Simply apologize and ask your partner to remind you if you have slipped again without noticing.

10. Let each other know how much you appreciate the fact that both of you are trying to make improvements in your communication. The subtext is that you care enough about each other and the integrity of your relationship to try to have dialogue flow as smoothly as possible. You are also admitting that some subjects are very difficult to talk about but that you will feel a lot better in the long run when you take communication risks with each other.

Tips for Arguing More Constructively and Fighting With Fairness

- Do not threaten your spouse or partner. If you do not recognize that you are threatening him or her, by all means apologize if he or she tells you that your choice of words, your tone of voice, or your nonverbal communication (e.g., shaking your finger, making a fist, staring, packing a suitcase) feels threatening.
- No name-calling: For example, "You're an idiot."
- Be specific and stay focused (as described above).
- Do not interrupt. Let your partner finish. However, it is incumbent on your partner not to go on and on so that you have no choice but to interrupt. So do not go on and on yourself. Be fair.
- If you and your partner or spouse are of different heights, do not argue standing up. Try being seated. It is very intimidating when someone taller than you is looking down on you.
- Watch your use of sweeping generalizations and absolutes such as, "You always leave the toilet seat up" or "You never initiate sex."
- Do not lecture your spouse or partner. Do not pontificate. Watch for stilted language. Apologize if you're confronted.
- You own your own feelings. Take responsibility for them.
- Be prepared to change one thing or many things about yourself. You will feel better for it and so will your relationship.

- Try not to lose perspective. Take a few deep breaths if necessary. Don't blow small issues inappropriately out of proportion.
- Give your spouse a chance to reflect on what he or she is feeling. Take a moment to reflect on what you are feeling too.
- Approach each argument with a solution as the goal. Watch for ulterior motives in yourself.
- Do not attack each other with strong verbal language, and do not attack each other physically. If you think that things are accelerating and getting out of control, take time out from each other for thirty minutes to an hour. Return to the argument later. However, you must return to it. You cannot sweep it under the carpet.
- Do not use arguments to dump all of your past hurts and resentments onto each other. This is not appropriate, and you will never resolve current conflicts by doing that.
- Be honest with each other, but also be gracious. There are both hurtful and less hurtful ways of talking about difficult issues. Try to be fair.
- Watch any tendency you might have to make assumptions about your partner. This is especially tempting and common if you have been together for a while. Ask your partner what he or she is thinking or feeling. Respond only to what is spoken, not what you assume is going on in your partner's mind or in your partner's heart. Try to change an attitude that one of you is right and one of you is wrong about the argument that you are having. Understand that each of you may perceive an event or recall a situation very differently. Do not continually defer to your partner's "better memory." You must compromise and you must try to meet each other halfway. Agreeing to disagree is perfectly acceptable.

Note

1. Some of the information in this chapter was adapted from *Messages: The Communication Skill Book* (McKay, Davis, & Fanning, 1983).

Reference

McKay, M., Davis, M., & Fanning, P. (1983). *Messages: The communication skill book.* Oakland, CA: New Harbinger.

4 Pay Attention to Life Cycle Issues

You will understand yourself and your partner or spouse a lot better if you pay some attention to the normal developmental issues for each of you as you go through life. If you are married, and have been for some time, you will be reassured to know that there are normal points of unrest and struggle common to almost all people in marriage. To appreciate and understand any marital conflict you are having, it is helpful to consider your stage of life and/or the stage of your marriage or other committed relationship. By respecting the stage-specific factors in yourself as an individual or in your relationship, you are less likely to blame yourself or your partner or spouse for all your difficulties. In a similar way, individuals may erroneously conclude that their relationship is pathological and should be ended when what is generating symptoms of relationship unrest is stage-specific.

Although we all pass through several stages from birth until death, I will describe only the stages relevant to the broad range of intimate relationships during medical training.

Stage 1: Early 20s

In this stage, you are in the process of becoming increasingly separate from your parents and becoming more independent. This includes for some of you leaving home to go to college and being away from home for eight or nine months of the calendar year. If you take summer employment away from your home community, you become even more accustomed to living on your own. For those of you who lived at home while attaining your undergraduate degree, you may be moving away from home for the first time when you begin medical

27

school. Although you may be still financially dependent on your family, you begin to feel increasingly psychologically independent. Should you become intimately involved with someone at this stage of life, you are simultaneously shifting allegiance and priority of connection from your family of origin to your partner. If you get married at this time and have been living at home until quite recently, you may find this shift quite challenging. In fact, you may feel caught in the middle between the needs and demands of your parents and those of your new spouse. Your parents and/or your parents-in-law may vary tremendously in their ability to be supportive and give you time and distance to adjust versus being controlling, interfering with your relationship, or both.

Stage 2: Late 20s

Many medical students will have graduated from medical school and will be considering residency or will be immersed in residency during this life stage. Because the course of study to become a physician takes so long, it is not unusual for medical students and residents at this life stage to still feel somewhat adolescent in their stage of maturity. Those of you who have had an earlier career before entering medical school would be exceptions to this because you have been living on your own and have also been financially independent before the age of 20 or in your early 20s. The major challenge or goal of Stage 2 is for you to become increasingly confident as a young professional while simultaneously becoming increasingly capable of intimacy. Disillusionment, however, is not uncommon; you may wonder if you have chosen the right partner or spouse. Periods of uncertainty may alternate with periods of clarity and conviction that you are happily committed. If you become a parent during this stage, you have the additional hurdle of adjusting to being a mother or father. You and your spouse both evolve into being a parent and observe each other as a mother and as a father. The challenge of being a parent may conflict with the time demands of your career of being a physician or any other engaging paid work outside the home. Striking a balance between one's commitment to work and one's commitment to family is often the biggest task of this stage of life.

Stage 3: Turning 30

Some of you will have been married or committed to somebody for around seven years at this point, and you may experience the "seven-year itch." If you are feeling particularly unhappy in your marriage, you may conclude that it is over and that you would do better with somebody else. Extramarital affairs are not uncommon at this age and stage of life. Some of you who are older medical students will be ready for commitment and marriage at this age (this could be a second marriage for some of you). The point of graduation from medical school is a turning point for many couples who have been together a few years. Some medical students get married at this time. Some get divorced.

Stage 4: The 30s

If you are in your 30s as a medical student and you are uncommitted, developing a relationship may be quite important to you. You may be also quite anxious to start a family. If you have been married for some time, you may be quite settled as a couple and may already have one or several children. This stage tends to be a settling-down stage of individual development. If your marriage is a good one, there should be a marked increase in your feelings of intimacy for each other; if your marriage is unhealthy, there may be gradual distancing from each other during these years.

These four stages are presented for guidance only. As I stated earlier, they enable individuals to better discern the way they are feeling about themselves as individuals as well as about each other. Many of you will be at very different stages of life when you enter medical school and when you graduate. Although the vast majority of you will be clustered in the mid-20s age range, some of you will be in your early 20s, and some will be in your late 30s. You are also members of an increasingly pluralistic group that brings unique and rich racial and ethnic diversity to these life stages.

Gender Differences

It may be helpful to explain some of the gender differences between men and women regarding marriage or other intimate relationships. Women tend to define themselves more in terms of their relationships with others. This helps to explain the concern with connection and communication that most women in marriage have. It is part of the historical caretaking function of women in marriage. This also accounts for the fact that most requests for marital help emanate from the woman in the relationship. Many men have extreme ambivalence about commitment and connection to someone in an intimate relationship. In other words, they both desire it and fear it. As part of normal male development, boys learn from an early age that healthy growth must often occur outside of relationships, outside of connection. They put much more time and emphasis on strength, independence and self-sufficiency, achievement, and supporting themselves. Although the situation is rarely addressed, when men get married, they usually feel much more competent at their work than they do at communication with their wives.

Why Get Married?

Ask yourself, Why do I want to get married? or, Why did I get married? Some of you will answer that you have a need, willingness, and capacity for intimacy with another person. You will understand that marriage is a commitment that you are making to one another and that you have the wish to share parts of yourselves with each other. Some of you will argue that your identity is quite stable; others that you are a work in progress. This is where your life stage at the time of marriage is quite critical. If you met each other when you were teenagers or in your early 20s and are now in your mid-20s, you will probably feel ready for marriage even though you may be in only the first or second year of medical school. Your good friends who are your age and in the same year of medical school, but who are not going out with anyone, may feel very different from you. They may feel completely uninterested in a commitment and value their state of being unattached with gusto.

Some of you will have married or will be getting married for a sense of security. This may be financial, physical, or psychological. Some of you may feel "incomplete without a partner or spouse." If you have come from an unhappy home, especially one in which you did not feel wanted or loved or were perhaps abused, you may have married to feel secure, loved, and fulfilled as a human being. It is important for you to remember, however, that marriage is not a panacea and that you must continue to work on your individual self-esteem and self-confidence and avoid becoming overly dependent on your spouse for your happiness and strength.

Some of you may have gotten married because you were pregnant or you had an urgent desire to have children. If at all possible, it is critical that both of you are at this stage of "generativity" together. You will have enormous conflicts with each other if one of you feels pressured into starting a family or getting married for this reason when you are not psychologically ready or interested. Don't forget that chronological age can be largely irrelevant. In other words, one of you feels that your biological clock is ticking, but the other doesn't at all.

Finally, some of you may have married for social reasons. In other words, you may have fallen victim to the societal rule and expectation that being married is normal and being single is not. Or some of you may have felt pressure from your families to get married. These ideas may sound ridiculous or anachronistic to many of you, but they are commonly felt by medical students and residents. It is not unusual for parents of women medical students to be simultaneously proud of their daughters and critical of them if they are not in a committed relationship or show much interest in being in one. The following statement or its equivalent is not uncommon: "You're not going to take that fellowship are you? Don't you think you're spending too much time and energy on your career and not enough time on your social life? Aren't you concerned that piling up all these degrees is going to work against you in the marriage market?" Male medical students and residents rarely hear these kinds of admonitions from their parents. We live in a very coupled society: Older medical students, residents, and practicing physicians who have never married, who are divorced, who are gay or lesbian and uncoupled, or who are widowed not uncommonly feel stigmatized. This seems to be a life cycle problem; that is, it's fine to be single until a certain age, but not fine after this arbitrary age and stage of life.

Case Examples

"My husband and I are both 30 years old. I'm graduating from medical school this year. We've been together for 10 years and married for eight. We have a son and a daughter who are seven and five years old. I don't think I want to be married any more. Could this be a stage that I'm going through?"

It's good that you are asking the question. It tells me that you are trying to understand your ambivalence or negative feelings about remaining married. It is interesting that this corresponds to your graduating from medical school and beginning the next chapter of your life. You may be wondering how common this feeling is in other graduating married medical students or in women who have been married the length of time that you have been. Or you are possibly looking for reassurance that what you are feeling is common or normal and that these feelings will pass once you graduate and begin your residency.

Let me ask you these questions, which I hope will help to explore what is happening. Think about your statement, "I don't think I want to be married any more." What are some of the reasons why you might be feeling this way? Does marriage feel like a responsibility that you no longer want? Are you interested in being a single woman again and being on your own? Does living alone or as a single parent with your children have some appeal to you? Have you ever lived on your own? Does the notion of not having to engage with a spouse appeal to you? Are you longing for some peace or quiet or down time? Are you interested in dating other men? How happy are you with your husband? Are you bored with him? Do you feel angry or resentful toward him? How vital is your marriage? Do you have fun together or share interests? What is your companionship like with him? Do you have enough independence of him? Do you get enough alone time in your marriage? How is your sexual relationship with your husband?

Here are some more questions: Are you depressed or unhappy or uncertain about things in your life? Would you like to be living somewhere else? How do you feel about your friends? Do you feel like you are putting in time or that you are in a rut? Are you irritable and easily angered with people? Are you excessively self-critical? Do you feel guilty a lot of the time? If you have answered in the affirmative to many of these questions, do not make a decision about your marriage right now. It is very important that you get the perspective of a trained professional regarding your mood. If you are depressed, you will be viewing many aspects of your life in a negative way. It would be inappropriate or premature to end your marriage if you have an unrecognized and untreated depression. You may view your marriage very differently when your mood is brighter.

Given your age and how long you've been together, you got married quite young. Do you feel that you've missed out on things? Do you regret that you have had quite a lot of responsibility from an early age and not enough fun? Looking back, do you feel that you dated enough or had much sexual experience before getting married? Do you envy women your age who do not have the responsibilities of marriage like you do?

Do you feel that you had enough time getting to know your husband before you started your family? Were your children planned, or did you find yourself pregnant before you were really ready to have kids? Did you have enough time together as a childless couple before starting your family?

You may or may not be going through a life stage issue—the age 30 transition. Let me offer the following suggestions:

• Start talking to your husband about the way you are feeling if you haven't done so already. He may feel the same way. If your husband has some of the feelings that you do but is not considering separation, he may have suggestions on how to deal with these feelings. It is possible that a dialogue between the two of you may help to clarify your feelings and facilitate more closeness and understanding between the two of you. This will be especially important if you or each of you has been feeling unloved, unappreciated, dismissed, distant, bored, or angry about things.

• You should talk with someone other than your husband about the way you are feeling. This could be a close friend, a classmate, a sibling, one or both of your parents, or a mentor in medicine. It's important, though, that the person you talk to is someone you respect for his or her listening ability, lack of judgment, trustworthiness, and maturity and wisdom. Opening up may help enormously. These feelings may pass, and this will allow you to navigate to a deeper level of acceptance of your life and your marriage.

• If your situation is really much more difficult than this or if you have a pervasive sense that you really are quite unhappy at home or if you feel depressed and trapped, I suggest that you get some professional help. You may benefit tremendously in speaking with someone with training, experience, and objectivity about what is happening to you and your marriage. This individual will assess you and provide guidance for you to explore options and solutions.

"My wife and I are both final-year medical students. We got married two years ago. Is it normal to feel disillusioned?"

Yes! There are a lot of myths attached to marriage, and one of them is that our spouses will be perfect and meet all of our needs and that we will then feel eternally happy, whole, and at peace. This is really in the realm of magical thinking and is, in part, a residue from childhood. It is not unlike the way we expected our parents to meet all of our needs and were furious at them when they didn't. All marriages can be stressful at times, extremely confusing, and intermittently so full of conflict and misunderstanding that one or both parties feel upset, disappointed, and hopeless. Therefore, it is not uncommon to ask questions such as, Did I make a mistake? Have I married the wrong person? Should I have gotten married at all? Perhaps there is somebody else out there who is better—someone who will love me unconditionally, who will make me feel more attractive, who will want more sex, who will want less sex, who will listen a lot better than my spouse, who will be less critical of me and more accepting of my shortcomings, who will be stronger and more independent, and so on and so on.

It is completely normal for you to have feelings of disillusionment that come and go during the early years of marriage. As you probably already know, they are extremely common when people are feeling tense with each other or are going through a difficult time together. Feeling discouraged and disillusioned is very common during or following an argument. If your feelings of disillusionment pass relatively quickly, especially after having a good talk with your wife, or making love, then there is really nothing to worry about. On the other hand, if your feelings of disillusionment have been going on for weeks or months, then something is wrong. Something is amiss that needs attention. You should talk about your feelings with your wife as well as with a close and trusted friend. If they still persist, you should talk with your family physician, your clergyman or clergywoman if you are religiously affiliated, or a psychotherapist.

Feelings of disillusionment can mean many things:

- This is a stage of life or a stage of marriage that is temporary and completely normal.
- You and your wife are having a lot of stress, and this stress is affecting your marriage.
- You may be experiencing some symptoms of depression.
- Disillusionment may be a symptom of marital trouble, and this calls for marital therapy.
- Your marriage may be in serious trouble and is no longer working.
- Your marriage was never really right in the first place, and you and your spouse are incompatible.
- You and your wife may need to separate and divorce.

My goal in this chapter has been an attempt to illustrate that all human beings have cycles and stages in their lives. These cycles and stages color our thoughts, feelings, hopes, and dreams regarding intimate relationships and marriage. As medical students, what preoccupies you and your spouse or partner and what you decide at this stage of life may be very different from what you do at another stage. It is much easier to see your way clear when you understand that a lot of the confusion and misunderstanding that you feel about yourself and each other is common, normal, or time limited.

5

Why Am I
So Miserable?

"Why am I so miserable?" These were Beth's words when she called to ask if she could come to see me about her marriage. Beth was a final-year medical student who had just completed an elective in ambulatory psychiatry when she called. Like most students, she didn't really have time to examine her marriage; she had been rotating through very busy services, on call one night in three, and preparing for examinations for months. Her husband Tom was a resident in general surgery. He too was very busy. They had been together since college and had been married since she was a first-year medical student. It was listening to her patients' stories in the outpatient psychiatry clinic that got Beth looking inward and prompted her rhetorical question, Why am I so miserable?

If this question applies to you, the first order of business is to ask yourself if you indeed feel this way or if you have been told by your partner or spouse that you are miserable. If it is the latter, have you come to believe it—that he or she is correct, that you are negative, irritable, critical, and no fun to be around? How do others find you? What do your friends, classmates, and family members say? If you do indeed feel miserable—irrespective of whether your partner or spouse notices or not—you are also saying, I don't like myself this way. Ask yourself these questions: Am I unhappy about school or about other things in my life? If so, is my upset and worry spilling over into my relationship and thereby concerning my partner or spouse—that I am contaminating our relationship with my misery?

What about asking the questions the other way around? That is, am I unhappy about my relationship? Is it my relationship that is making me feel miserable? Am I unhappy with my partner or spouse? Am I bored? Lonely? Do I feel trapped in this relationship? Did I get married (or get committed) too young? Or too quickly? Do I feel envious of my single friends who don't have

35

the responsibility that I do, who have more independence, who don't have to share with or accommodate to anyone, who can do whatever or move anywhere they would like? Am I grieving? Am I sad about hopes and dreams that I attached to this relationship that just aren't happening or will never happen—that my partner or spouse is not who I thought and I'm filled with disappointment and regret.

What Do I Do?

First, discuss your situation with your partner or spouse. Has he or she noticed that you're not feeling very well? Does he or she feel similar to the way that you are feeling? You may find that just talking together about this helps a bit—or a lot! Why?

• You are getting something "off your chest," and that in itself feels like a relief. It can feel very isolating and heavy to bear such strong worries all alone; hence, just ventilating can make you feel lighter. And if any of your perceptions or ideas are wrong or distorted, they may be corrected by input from your partner or spouse.

• You are unclogging communication blockages that may have been in place but that were not really obvious to you—or to your partner. Your awareness of something being freed up in your talk with each other will be welcome and overdue if it has been a long time since you have had such a good talk or if you have never spoken so frankly to each other. It may be that you are literally bursting with bottled up energy and emotion. Your busyness may have actually been a way of avoiding recognition that communication hasn't been flowing easily between the two of you. So what has appeared as a cause of lack of time together is actually the result of something else.

• You are learning about the dynamics of your relationship as you speak and gaining more understanding about yourself and your partner. Listening to your words and feelings, especially if they are raw, disorganized, and coming from deep within, can tell you a lot about yourself "in relation"—that is, in a committed relationship to someone with whom you feel vulnerable and perhaps fearful, fearful of his or her response or lack of response to you. Remember that every relationship is unique and ever evolving. By talking like this, you are charting a new course together, for better or for worse.

• You will change in some way, as will your partner, as a result of this talk together. You may find that your ideas are way off base and that they will be corrected by his or her responses. You may find that your concerns and fears are not groundless, that there are very serious issues that the two of you are facing.

Second, discuss your situation with a friend or with a member of your family with whom you are close. This helps to reduce the aloneness that you may be feeling about your situation. If you are fairly new to the community where you are living and have not made a good friend yet, someone you can really trust, you may need to call a friend who lives away. It will be worth the telephone call!

Male medical students, please note: It may be harder for you to reach out to a friend, but work at it. Men in general tend to be more self-reliant, independent, and closed about such deeply personal matters. This has been called the white knight complex (Dickstein, 1986) and it tends to mask inner feelings of need for others and normal dependency. You will feel better for speaking to someone you trust and respect—and this kind of talk will also strengthen your friendship. Some men find it easier to talk to a female friend than to a male friend. If you have the luxury, speak to both; a gender perspective may or may not be helpful, depending on the specifics of your situation.

Male and female medical students, please note: If you feel threatened by having your partner or spouse talk to someone about your relationship, say so! This isn't uncommon—to feel exposed, critiqued, or even betrayed about something as intimate as your relationship. And this will be even more so depending on the specifics that you know or imagine will be talked about, especially personal problems that are causing relationship strain: Are you struggling academically? Do you have an eating disorder? Are you drinking too much? Do you have sexual difficulties? Are you confused about your sexual orientation? Are you having an affair with someone? Are you a battered spouse? The list is endless. You have a right to privacy, but your partner also has the right to receive support. What is key is the character of the friend in whom your partner or spouse confides. Is he or she someone with integrity, maturity, and respect for confidentiality?

Third, discuss your situation with a therapist. Unlike a friend, a professional with training in human relations will be able to bring a blend of objectivity and sensitivity to your situation that should help you. By listening carefully to you and using a diagnostic lens, a therapist should be able to sift through all of the factors making you feel so unhappy and confused. Most important, you will feel validated and affirmed that what you are feeling is very real and understandable given the circumstances of your relationship. Another question that will be answered is how much your misery is a result of relationship problems and how much is the cause—or both. And whether or not you alone need treatment or whether the two of you do.

Hilary was referred to me through the Student Health Office of our university where she was majoring in anthropology. The primary care physician had diagnosed her with depression and wanted her to take an antidepressant. She was reluctant to begin medication without the opinion of a psychiatrist. Her husband, Warren, was a final-year medical student. He had been my student in third year, and he wanted his wife to be assessed by me. What I found was this: Yes, she was depressed but not clinically depressed. She was very angry—and understandably. She and Warren were both full-time students, yet she was doing virtually everything to run and maintain the home. So she was exhausted and felt used—and guilty for complaining. Her husband argued that he had to study much harder than her, that medicine was a calling and more important than her studies, and that in their culture, housework was her job, not his. He would soon be earning "big money," and she would be compensated for her hard work. Her mother agreed with her husband. Her aunt, a physician married to another physician, told her, "Medicine is not a 9-to-5 job; get used to it. You will have to always do 75% of the work at home if you want your marriage to succeed." I took a very different approach. I invited her husband to come in the next time with her. I explained the importance of fairness in marriage and that his ideas about medical work being more important than her work and studies were not true and were self-serving—which he accepted. I also helped the two of them to negotiate a more equitable distribution of household duties and responsibilities, which they did with mutual respect and love. In no time, Hilary was feeling better, and so was he. "It's great to come home to a happy person again!"

Reference

Dickstein, L. J. (1986). Social change and dependency in university men: The white knight complex unresolved. *Journal of College Student Psychotherapy, 1*, 31-41.

6 We're a Gay Couple

The profession of medicine has come a long way in the last generation or two in recognizing and accepting that a certain percentage of medical students are gay or lesbian. Contemporary medical students who are open about their homosexuality generally feel a high level of acceptance by their medical school peers. They are less certain, however, about their professors and attending physicians. It is easier to be an openly gay or lesbian medical student in cities such as New York or San Francisco than it is in states such as Mississippi or parts of the Midwest, and irrespective of geographical location, it is less common to be open about your gayness if you are attending a medical school that is religiously affiliated.

If you are a gay or lesbian medical student, you are probably just as interested in a close and loving relationship with one particular person as your heterosexual counterparts. The wish for a steady and intimate relationship, now or later, is part of the human condition and has nothing to do with sexual orientation. Similarly, if you are a member of a gay or lesbian couple, your challenges are much more similar to heterosexual couples than they are different. All medical student couples, irrespective of sexual orientation, are prone to problems with balancing work, study, and family; overworking; communicating; making love; coping with illness in themselves or family members; struggling with finances; and so forth.

Those of you who are familiar with the struggles for gay rights in North America or who have mentors who have fought those battles will know that they have not been easily won. Domestic partnerships now enjoy some measure of protection of assets and property rights, custody rights, health and pension benefits, and other legal issues. Some of you have had or will have commitment ceremonies. Unfortunately, segments of our society remain passionately antihomosexual, and you will find that in some communities, gay and lesbian physicians and their partners cannot live openly with acceptance

39

and dignity. Given how tough it is for intimate relationships to succeed in our society, the psychological significance of this basic attitudinal difference toward gay and lesbian couples, as opposed to heterosexual couples, cannot be underestimated.

Let me turn now to some of the unique issues for gay and lesbian medical students in intimate relationships.

Gay Male Medical Student Couples

Intimacy

For many gay men, building and maintaining intimacy with another man can be a dance. In other words, as much as you long for and want intimacy with someone, you are at the same time frightened of it and pushing the other person away. I have heard many men, both gay and straight, who describe how easy it is for them to be sexual with their partners, but they have much more difficulty with intimacy. Physical attraction leads to erotic feelings within themselves as well as erotic signals from their partners, and this leads to exploration and sexual involvement. When men discuss difficulty with intimacy, they are usually talking about a sense of discomfort and difficulty with connection with intense and deep feelings for another and with committing themselves to that person in an exclusive and mutually respectful way. Furthermore, it is not unusual for men to have skewed ideas about the meaning of a committed relationship. They confuse commitment with dependence and entrapment, which is pretty frightening. A healthy relationship has a nice balance of autonomy and intimacy. You must talk about your feelings with your partner; resist the temptation to solve complicated and confusing feelings in the bedroom. In fact, the vast majority of sexual difficulties that occur in gay male couples are not physical or mechanical; they are invariably due to unexpressed feelings between the two individuals.

Coming Out

If you and your partner are both at the same stage of coming out, you are fortunate because you will be well matched in the barriers that you have put behind you and the ones that you are yet to face. Furthermore, there will be a resonance and a deep understanding of any resistance that each of you has toward disclosing your sexual orientation to others. If one of you is much further along in accepting your homosexuality and if you have done a lot of disclosure to your family and close friends, you may have difficulty fully appreciating your partner's inertia if he is confused about his sexual orientation, ambivalent about it, and quite closeted. It is very important that you be sympathetic and patient. This is a tall order—a tall order because if you have spent years coming to the point where you are, you will not want to feel stuck or perhaps that you are being forced back into the closet. If your partner feels that he might be bisexual, make sure that you let him know how much that scares you—that is, that he may abandon you and seek out a female partner instead. If your partner is unambivalently gay but is excessively private by your estimation, your support and role modeling should help him to slowly and selectively come out to the important people in his life.

Competition

Because you are both men, you may have some difficulties competing with each other. Remember that men are socialized to be independent, self-sufficient, strong, and competitive. Competition in medical students is not unusual, given how much you had to compete with others academically to be admitted to medical school in the first place. It is very difficult to "turn off" being competitive once you receive the letter of acceptance to medical school. Some branches of medicine are more competitive than others, and you may witness situations in your medical training in which professors and attending physicians foster competition in their trainees. Some of this could or may spill over into your personal intimate relationship life.

What are some of the other areas in which you and your partner may compete? Money may be one of them, although most medical students don't have much money. However, you may aspire to branches of medicine that are more highly remunerative, or you may come from a monied family. Or your partner may have more money than you. How much money a man has can be one of the regulators of his self-esteem. Intelligence is another area of competition. Men like to prove how smart they are with each other, and again, in certain branches of medicine, one-upmanship is very common. If you and your partner seem to be arguing or competing about matters relating to intelligence, it is very important to address it and explore your feelings with each other. Other areas of competition include the following: how handsome you are, how athletic you are or gifted at sports, how popular you are, how good you are in bed (sexual prowess), how well you cook, or how highly developed your taste is in art or design.

As you can see, these areas of competition are the surface manifestation of something deeper. If they go unaddressed, you can have a relationship with lots of tension, arguing, and distancing from each other. If each of you looks inward and talks about what you see, you should be able to have a frank and wholesome discussion about themes that could be affecting each of you—for example, self-esteem, self-acceptance, trust, commitment, and how secure you feel in the relationship.

Having Sex Outside Your Relationship

During the gay liberation movement and before herpes and AIDS, many committed gay couples had sexually open relationships. In most circles, this model is anachronistic today. Gay men feel most comfortable and most secure with monogamy. That said, you need to watch for sexual acting out in yourself and in your partner. Sexual acting out is most apt to occur when men do not face their difficulties head on. In other words, you need to work at recognizing and talking about your feelings of unhappiness, loneliness, resentments, and slights. My advice is simple: Talk about what is going on in your heart and in your soul. Don't go cruising for sex with strangers. It's like the song "Looking for Love in All the Wrong Places." It's not worth the risk. Here is an example of sexual acting out involving a medical student.

> Dr. I. and Dr. J., both residents, came to see me in the midst of a huge relationship crisis. Dr. I. came home from work one day and confessed that he was having an affair with a medical student on his service. Dr. J. was horrified, not only because his relationship was in jeopardy but also because of the ethical issues associated with supervisor-trainee dynamics (although both Dr. I. and his student were trainees, Dr. I. was supervising the student and evaluating him for the program director). I learned very quickly that there were lots of reasons why the relationship was strained and Dr. I. was vulnerable: They were a closeted couple (Dr. I. was in orthopedics and Dr. J. was in urology), so they had very few external supports. They each were on call a lot and could not always coordinate their schedules, so they didn't see each other very often. Although they had a good sexual relationship, neither communicated feelings of love, tenderness, vulnerability, or insecurity very easily. Dr. I. was on probation, and this made him feel very second rate and ashamed—feelings he'd never shared with Dr. J. After two conjoint visits in which I was able to get these two men talking to each other again—and with more honesty and mutual sensitivity than ever before—Dr. I. ended the rela-

tionship with his student. This young man, fortunately, accepted this decision with grace and with no fallout at work or reporting to the program director.

Difference in Age

If there is a major difference in age between you and your partner, this may not be a problem for the two of you, but it may be problematic for your family or friends. You actually might find your relationship quite complementary. In other words, if you are the younger person, you may be attracted to the wisdom of your partner, his maturity, or his financial stability. He in turn may be attracted to your appearance, your youth, your openness, and your promise. But remember you are at different stages of the male life cycle. If you are the younger partner and do not become as self-sufficient or self-fulfilled as your partner expects, you may find him overly controlling and dominating of you. Also, be sure to tell him if you find him possessive and jealous of your friendships with men your own age.

AIDS

With advanced knowledge about transmission of HIV and important public health measures, fewer medical students are infected with HIV than a decade or two ago. But if you are an older medical student or if your partner is an older man, your lives may have been intimately touched by colleagues or friends living with or who have died of HIV-AIDS. When one or both partners are HIV positive, most relationship symptoms are due to loss—loss of health and physical livelihood, companionship, work, independence, privacy, financial security, sexual intimacy, self-esteem, and with severe disease progression, personal dignity. Fortunately, with newer antiretroviral drugs (especially the protease inhibitors), HIV-positive individuals are not only living longer but also enjoying a much higher quality of life.

Being a Gay Father

Once again, if you are an older gay medical student, you may have one or more children from a previous relationship. You will have the same challenges as other divorced or blended families if your former wife has remarried. There is a stepfather now for your children, resulting sometimes in confusion and uncertainty over roles and responsibilities. If you are coupled, do not be surprised if your children are threatened by your partner. They—both your children *and*

your partner—may compete for your love and attention. You will have to decide whether or not the true nature of your relationship with your partner is disclosed to your children or not—and if so, how private you wish to be about this
matter. Some children who have a gay father are out with their friends, and
some are not.

Lesbian Medical Student Couples

Achieving a Balance of
Interdependence and Independence

A not uncommon struggle of women in a lesbian relationship is developing
a comfort level on the interdependence-independence continuum. You may
need to do a fair amount of talking and negotiating about this matter to feel
comfortable. It is absolutely essential that you protect your sense of individual-
ity and your ability to continue to socialize with other women and men. Jeal-
ousy, overdependence, and high levels of insecurity in either one of you are not
healthy for your relationship.

Coming Out

In general, accepting oneself as a lesbian woman in North American society
is not quite as difficult as it is for gay men. Internalized homophobia—that is,
one's inner sense of anxiety about or negative feelings about homosexuality—
tends to be much higher in men than in women. If you and your partner are at
the same stage of accepting and disclosing your sexual orientation, that makes
it much easier to declare your couplehood and to receive love and support from
your family, friends, and colleagues. However, if one of you is "into settling
down" but the other is "needing her freedom," this will be a problem.

Sexual Difficulties

No problem here if both you and your partner have the same interest in sex
and the forms that your love-making take with each other. Lots of lesbian couples are no longer erotic with each other but share a very high level of physical
affection. If you have a history of having been sexually abused as a girl or sexually assaulted as a young woman, you may be suffering emotional conse-
quences of this. And even though you are now involved in a lesbian relationship, you may still have difficulties with trust, have wobbly self-esteem, have

difficulty becoming sexually aroused or experiencing orgasms, or have a lot of anxiety in general along with phobic symptoms specific to intimate relationships. You should consider individual, and possibly couples, therapy. You will find it very helpful.

Being a Lesbian Mother

You or your partner may have a child or children that you brought into this relationship or who are from this relationship. There are lots of different situations. You or your partner may have been married before and have a child or children by that marriage. Or one of you might have had a consensual sexual relationship with a male friend for the sole purpose of conception. You and your partner or previous partner may have a child by artificial insemination or other types of reproductive technology. Or the two of you may have adopted a child. Hopefully, you are living in a progressive community and your same-sex family receives the same rights, recognition, and support as other families in your neighborhood. And if you are part of a stepfamily, hopefully there are no problems with your partner's ex-husband and custody and access of your shared children.

Issues Around Separation

If you and your partner are separating, and especially if the two of you have children, consider getting some therapy. Separation can be really tough going in the early weeks and months, and if you are fortunate to have a good support group, this will ease the passage. However, this societal support is not always as forthcoming as it is when heterosexual people are separating, and this could contribute to a sense of isolation or loneliness. If you are lucky to be studying in a city with a good-sized lesbian community, it will be easier for you to be on your own, as well as to meet other women without intruding on your ex-partner's personal space.

Here is an example of a lesbian couple struggling with some of these issues.

Cheryl and Marilyn came to see me when Cheryl was in first-year medical school and Marilyn was in her final year of architecture. Cheryl started: "I'm here because we're becoming more and more serious about each other, and quite frankly, I'm scared of that." Marilyn said, "I'm here because Cheryl wants this—counseling. I don't really think we need it; we're big people. But if it helps us, I'm all for it. Cheryl says I overpower her, that she isn't always straight with me, that I shut her down, which I find kind of funny because everyone in my family thinks I'm a wimp—which is true. I come from a rather tough, aggressive bunch of go-getters." They were both 22 years old. In therapy, they wanted to work on trying to decide whether to live together or not, learning to communicate more effectively, improving their sexual relationship, making more couple friends, and helping Cheryl to come out to her family.

I asked more questions about the two of them and learned that this was the first serious relationship for each. But they were at different stages of coming out. Cheryl had never really spent any time with other lesbians; the two of them had met at a college basketball tournament and became friendly. Cheryl had dated men until about two years earlier when she came to accept that she was lesbian. Marilyn, however, had come out in high school and was very open with her family and friends. She had dated a few other women but nothing serious until meeting Cheryl. I highlighted their different positions on the coming-out axis so that they would both understand that this can, and often does, explain miscommunication and misunderstanding in relationships.

I also explained that their temperaments were very different. Cheryl was rather shy, reserved, and private. Marilyn was much more extroverted and direct. I emphasized the complementary nature of their attraction to each other—and that, for the most part, it worked! I also pointed out that the same differences that were appealing to one another were occasionally the things that they recoiled from. They reflected a lot on that common dynamic in couples.

We talked a lot about sex. And I came to know that they had different wishes, likes, and dislikes. Their attitudes were wholesome and healthy. The problem was in talking about it. Again, Cheryl preferred to be indirect, allusive, suggestive, and mysterious. She was also quite romantic. Marilyn was blunt and "in your face" but no less romantic. She liked to tease and shock. They did manage to find a compromise and to laugh more both in the bedroom and outside it.

Discussions about living together were very fruitful. In the end, they decided not to live together, and this felt mutually OK. But at first, it was hard for Marilyn; she really wanted to set up house together. Despite her age, she really wanted to settle down—perhaps because she was graduating and Cheryl was just starting medical studies. But also, Marilyn had been on her own a lot since she was 17. Cheryl had not; she'd lived at home while getting her undergraduate degree. She really liked living alone, having her own space, and not having to share. She was candid: "I take living together very seriously. I'm just not ready."

As the weeks went on, Cheryl became increasingly open with her classmates about her relationship with Marilyn. Together, they attended a number of medical school social events. They also met some other couples—both gay and straight. Cheryl decided to come out to her mother (her father was dead); that went quite well, overall, and Marilyn helped enormously. Cheryl's mom was very comfortable with Marilyn and liked her a lot; they shared a similar spunky nature—and they both played jazz piano!

The subtext of my therapy with the two of them was acceptance of their relationship. My belief in them was helpful, I think—as well as the assistance I provided toward their talking with each other more effectively. This involved bringing out Cheryl more, pointing out when she was being passive-aggressive, and helping Marilyn to be more tactful in her approach to Cheryl. They worked hard between sessions on their difficulties, and they did very well.

7 You Never Want to Make Love Anymore!

"You never want to make love anymore!" Sounds accusatory, doesn't it? Well, it is. Is this true? It's your perception, so you'd better check it out with your spouse or partner. How might he or she respond to this?

- "Go to hell!"
- (sarcastically) "And you're such a hot number yourself."
- "Funny, I was just thinking the same thoughts about you! I've been feeling pretty rejected by you too."
- "Not true. I do feel like making love . . . sometimes . . . occasionally . . . but not as often as you do I guess, given the tone of your words."
- "Not true. I always feel like making love—but I rarely feel like just having sex—that is, having sex as we have it, as we do it. It's not very enjoyable for me. I think we need to talk about it."
- "Almost true. I rarely want to have sex, make love, whatever you want to call it, anymore. Why? Because our relationship is so worn down and we're both so resentful and so distant with each other. There's no intimacy. Most of the time, I feel that you despise me. You're always angry at me. How am I supposed to feel good about making love with you? No thanks! And no mercy sex either please."
- "True. I haven't wanted to make love in ages. Our relationship is dead. I want out. I don't love you anymore."

All of these responses will lead to more discussion, which is what this topic needs in your relationship. However, let me suggest a better way than "You never want to make love anymore!" Drop the *never*. It's too absolute. And this word, plus the assuming tone of your question, is very provocative. How about something like, "Can we talk about our sex life? . . . I perceive . . . or my sense is . . . that you don't feel like making love with me much these days. Is that so?" Or how about talking about your feelings—that is, how you feel about your love life these days: "I'm really worried about our sexual relationship. I feel like making love. . . . I want to get closer again. When we don't make love I feel scared . . . down . . . lonely . . . ripped off . . . tense. I really miss the closeness we used to have. Can we talk about it?"

How Do You Talk About Sex?

Don't assume that because you are a medical student or someone who has studied anatomy, sexual physiology, psychology, or reproductive health that you should be well versed in discussing your sexual life with your partner or spouse. That is a myth. Medical students, physicians, and other health professionals have as much difficulty with their sex lives as any group. We are human. Ultimately, recognizing and talking about something as personal as one's sexual feelings is very challenging in the midst of an intimate relationship. Why? Because in no other relationship are we as vulnerable, naked, and subject to being wounded. It is easy to become defensive very quickly—even before the subject is broached. No wonder many people in intimate relationships avoid talking together about their sex life.

Pick the right time—or a sort of right time—to bring up the subject. There is no real right time, but some times are better than others. You will have learned when the wrong times are to discuss with each other difficult or potentially difficult topics. So avoid those moments. And just launch into it.

Try to discuss foreplay with each other: Is there enough of it? How much begins long before you ever touch each other—by thought, words, and affectionate acts? How much nonsexual affection is there—touching, holding hands, hugging, kissing each other? How much sexual affection is there—touching in an erotic way of each other's anatomy? Penis, clitoris, breasts, nipples, buttocks, and so on? Oral versus manual stimulation? Do either of you have any problems with arousal—that is, with lubrication or erections? What about orgasm—frequency, intensity, simultaneously versus sequentially? Is this satisfactory to both of you? Does either one of you feel rushed? Does either one of you feel unauthentic? That is, you are faking that you are interested, excited, or having an orgasm because you feel you "should" or "it's your duty" or "it's been two weeks. . . . I'd better get it over with" or "I'd better do it to keep him or her happy"?

The above paragraph is a very bare-bones sketch of a few of the things to try to talk about with each other. For some of you, this will appear rather elementary. For others, it will be quite a hurdle. What is key is the openness and willingness of each of you to try to discuss a deeply sensitive and personal matter with forethought, sensitivity, delicacy, trust, and love. Some individuals and couples like to browse through popular books and manuals on sex to facilitate their talk with each other; others find them a barrier or too intimidating.

What About *Not* Talking About Sex?

You may not have a sex problem, but you may have a problem with your relationship, especially with closeness, that has resulted in a change in your sexual life together—a breakdown in the sexual expression of your love for each other. So what you need to talk about is the two of you.

Respect

How much do you respect your partner, your husband, your wife? What parts of him or her do you respect more than others? Are you sitting on anger or resentment that may be blocking your affection for each other? Do you feel respected by your partner or spouse? If not, have you talked about it? You must, if you haven't. You have a responsibility to him or her to be honest and forward with those feelings. If you believe that you have tried to discuss it but get nowhere and merely make your spouse defensive and argumentative, then that in a way proves your point, that you do not feel respected for owning those feelings. The most common responses to the statement: "I don't feel that you respect me" are one or more of the following:

- Shock: "I'm stunned. I *do* respect you."
- Shame: "I don't know what to say. I feel embarrassed."
- Defensiveness: "You're wrong—absolutely and completely wrong. I pride myself on how much I respect you. I'm better than most husbands (or wives)."
- Attack: "You're pathetic. You wouldn't know respect if it was staring you in the face."
- Sarcasm: "You're right. I forgot that you're the world authority on respect in marriage. I'm so fortunate to be the recipient of your omnipresent respect for me."

A much better response is this: "Yikes . . . I didn't know that you felt that way. Let's talk about it." By responding like this, you are showing respect and interest in understanding and trying to correct that feeling, to make it go away. Your response is an invitation toward engagement with your partner and your willingness to go deeper than statements and allegations such as, "You never want to make love anymore."

Trust

How do you talk about trust—and the role that it might be playing in your sexual difficulty? Bold statements such as, "I don't trust you anymore"; "You have betrayed my trust"; "There is no trust anymore in this relationship" are obviously indicative of a serious assault on or erosion of the basic regard in marriage. But problems with trust may not always be so gravely altered. What follows are not uncommon examples that I have gleaned from my work with medical student couples, examples that have affected sexual expression in the relationship or marriage:

- "I don't trust you anymore. You have lied to me so many times now that I have to question every word or action on your part."

- "Since you slept with Jennifer how can I trust you? Do you think I'm a fool?"

- "Telling Frank that I was seeing a psychiatrist really pisses me off. I'll never trust you again."

- "It's a whole series of little things—the way you put me down or make fun of my accent, the way you tease me about my dancing, the comments about my dad and his drinking, your comments about my grammar. That's why I don't trust you."

- "I do trust you with things on the surface. Like, I know you'll bring home a pay-check, that you will never hit me, that you love the kids, that you're a hard worker, but I would never trust you with my feelings. You just don't get it—how much you have hurt me."

- "Your eating disorder does strange things to my head—and to our marriage. Sorry to have to be so cruel, but I just don't trust you."

- "Let me explain it one last time. I have no interest in watching pornographic videos with you—and I'm not being a prude. I find them very threatening that you prefer those 'women' to me. I just can't trust you, David, like I used to. Sorry."

The key to restoring trust is talking to each other. Over and over again—until it feels that clearing the air and identifying hurts and misunderstandings allow defenses to yield a little and some good faith to surface. And tincture of time—time helps tremendously.

Romance

Romancing each other and feeling romanced are the bedrock of healthy sexual functioning in marriage. The everyday lives of people today, including medical students and their partners or spouses, are very busy. Unless you are in the early weeks and months of a courtship when sexual feelings are most immediate and often expressed, you will not be able to simply turn your erotic feelings for each other off and on like a switch. Romance is essential and really is the precursor to foreplay or (in some conceptualizations of sexual arousal) is the first step in foreplay. Romance is not taught in academic centers. It is not part of the core curriculum. It certainly is not taught in medical school. Indeed, some would argue that romance, because of its connection to physicians' personal lives, is drilled out of the training of doctors—that their solo or primary focus must be clinical training and that their personal lives must go on hold or simply flourish independently. We have not evolved as a discipline to the point of trainees' giving a Grand Rounds with a title such as "Restoring Romance With Your Spouse After Being on Call for 36 Hours: A Review of the Literature." We do not have medical journals with titles such as the *American Journal of Medicine and Marriage*. We do not regularly hear attending physicians telling their trainees, "Read up on juvenile diabetes for next Wednesday's seminar, but make sure that you spend part of the weekend hanging out with your wife/husband/partner, because I'm going to quiz you on that as well."

Suggestions

- Protect time to simply be together.
- Take turns shopping for and preparing a special meal to have together.
- Buy some candles.
- Even if you have had a terrible or a tiring day, always try to give each other a cheery greeting, which includes a kiss and a hug, before you ask, "How was your day?"
- Try to get out together once a week (or certainly once every two weeks) on a date. Even going for a walk and stopping at a cafe counts. And it's not expensive.
- If you have children, budget for a babysitter, or join a babysitting pool with other married students who are parents.
- Become liberal with compliments. Work at this if you are shy or reserved: "You look terrific today." "You're the handsomest guy in your class." "I'm so lucky you're in my life." "Hi gorgeous."
- Use lots of humor and tease each other. Watch for sarcasm, though.

- Send each other e-mails frequently; they can be brief. Leave messages on each other's voice mail and answering machines. Write affectionate words to each other on Post-it notes.

- Go to the university gym together, or run or cycle or swim together. Respect each other's different level of fitness and interest. Don't try to compete with each other unless it is wholesome and clean.

- Try to find one activity or hobby that you both enjoy doing together. This may take some brainstorming and experimenting, but don't give up.

- Women, if you have had children, accept the changes in your body. And to all husbands or partners, you too!

- Go dancing together.

- Spend a few minutes on a regular basis reading poems to each other.

- If you're worried about your sexual relationship, go to the library or to a bookstore and pick out one or more books *together.* It is absolutely critical that this be a shared experience and not an activity that one of you forces on the other. The spirit and context have to be right—a spirit of love and a context of mutuality.

What About Couples Therapy?

Here are two examples of people who came for couples therapy and gained from that experience.

Chad's chief complaint to Melinda was, "You never want to make love anymore." Melinda's chief complaint to Chad was, "Not true. I do want to make love, but not the way that you insist on making love. You won't listen to me about what I like and don't like." Chad continued, "It's very simple, Dr. Myers; Melinda won't let me stimulate her manually at all during foreplay. She keeps saying 'no' and pushing my hand away. I get really pissed off. What's weird is that she's fine with oral sex, which we both enjoy, but she hates manual sex. I don't know what I'm doing wrong. I'm real gentle, and I don't rush it, but she just won't have it." I invited Melinda to reply: "Chad's right. This drives him bananas, but he just won't take 'no' for an answer. If we don't get some help with this, I'm afraid we'll end up apart. I really love you Chad but I can't go on like this." The two of them argued about this for some time until I shifted away from their concerns and obtained general history about their relationship. They had met three years earlier when they were both first-year medical students. After a year of dating, they began living together. In all other respects, their relationship seemed to be functioning well. But this issue over sex was causing lots of upset. Chad was getting more angry and more irritable about it, and Melinda was becoming increasingly turned off about making love because of Chad's "obsessiveness" and sensitivity.

My individual visits with each of them were key: Melinda's background was chaotic. Her parents were both alcoholic. Her mother left the family when she was five and died a few years later, possibly of suicide. Her father began "touching" her shortly after her mother left the home, and this continued until she was 12. He was also physically violent with her younger brother, and Melinda submitted to her father's touching to distract her father from hitting her brother. All of this ended when her father accepted treatment for his alcoholism, and he never drank again. Because of years of sexual abuse, Melinda hated manual stimulation of her clitoral/vaginal area. Even Chad's interest in this made her very tense, panicky, or withdrawn. She decided never to tell Chad about her father's abuse because the two of them had a very good relationship. They played golf together and seemed to really like each other.

Chad's background was quite different: His mother was a physician and his father a businessman. They were comfortably middle class, and he did well academically and in sports. However, he was quite shy, and Melinda was his first girlfriend. He told me that he felt sexually inexperienced compared with Melinda because she had had several boyfriends before and had lived with one for a year in college. "That's why I want our sex life to be perfect. I want Melinda to feel as satisfied with me as she can possibly be. I want to make up for all the years she was having sex and I wasn't. I don't want to give her any reason for leaving me."

So what did I do to help? In my next few conjoint visits with the two of them, I told Chad that some people, both men and women, just don't enjoy manual sex. That that's normal and all human beings are different. I played up the positives in their relationship, especially all other aspects of their sexuality together that worked well and that gave each of them pleasure. I requested that he just try to put aside "touching" Melinda and enjoy what works so well in the bedroom. With this, Melinda felt much more relaxed with him so that their affection and sexual fulfillment soared. Quite spontaneously, Chad began to tell Melinda about his underlying sexual insecurities and his fear that she would become sexually disappointed in him. Melinda responded with surprise and compassion. She told him that never in her life had she ever felt so respected and loved, nor had she ever experienced such tender or passionate lovemaking.

*   *   *

Bill and Lara were on the verge of breaking up when they came for help. Bill was a second-year medical student, and Lara was a pharmacist. Lara was five months pregnant, and they were about to be married. Lara spoke first: "There's something abnormal about Bill. He's completely shut down sexually. We haven't made love in months. What's wrong with me? Am I that much of a turnoff? Should we be getting married with our sex life this bad?" She continued along this line with many plaintive rhetorical questions until I interrupted. Bill looked very distraught, and I wanted to hear from him. He spoke deliberately and very slowly. He didn't really look at me, nor did he look at Lara: "I think Lara is right. I am kind of pathetic. I don't think we should be here. I think that we should cancel the wedding and Lara should . . . should . . . just try to forget about me . . . and follow her own path." I said to myself, "This poor guy is very depressed." I steered away from their sexual relationship and asked some general questions of each of them. That helped a bit. Lara calmed down and Bill picked up a tiny bit. Thinking that Bill perhaps felt trapped into marriage because of the pregnancy, I explored that. No, both of them actually felt OK about becoming parents—initially. But as time went on, Bill seemed to shut down.

My individual visit with Lara was uneventful. She was very committed to Bill and was deeply worried about him. Bill's visit with me was heartbreaking. Not only was he genetically vulnerable to depression (both his mother and maternal grandmother had been treated for depression), but he was psychologically vulnerable, too. With great anguish and shame, Bill told me that he had been gang raped five years earlier while out of school for a year working as a logger. He and three other men had been out drinking. One of them had some marijuana, which they all smoked. Bill felt stoned like he had never felt before. When they returned to the cabin late at night, the other men turned on him, held him down, gagged him, and took turns sodomizing him. He had told no one before. Like so many male victims of sexual assault, Bill felt sexually dirty, violated, depressed, angry, fearful of men, insecure about his masculinity, and now confused about his sexual orientation. "Maybe I am gay. Maybe I wanted to be raped. Maybe I asked for it. Maybe I don't want to be a husband . . . or a dad."

What did I do? I told the two of them that I wanted to work with Bill in individual therapy and leave the couples treatment for now. They were both fine with this. I treated Bill also with an antidepressant medication, and we met for weekly psychotherapy for about a year. They canceled their wedding. Lara gave birth to a beautiful and healthy son, Adam, and she and Bill got married when Adam was six months old. Bill told Lara about the sexual assault and talked very openly with her about his therapy with me. She was very supportive and sensitive to the trauma he had experienced. Their sexual relationship returned and remained frequent and enjoyable, much like it was when they first met. Bill's therapy, his enhanced intimacy with Lara, their good sexual relationship, and his being a father to Adam all gave him a consolidated sense of being a healthy mature man. His thoughts of being gay ended with his healing.

All You Ever Want to Do Is Study. That's Hardly My Idea of Foreplay!

Is this true? Or is it more that you feel you *have to* study—to do well, to learn a good portion of the prescribed material, to pass your exams, to graduate? Are there some specific goals that you have by studying? Are you competing for awards and prizes for academic excellence? Are you trying to maintain a standard of achievement that is characteristic of you since childhood or adolescence that has now become an imperative in your life? Are you used to being the best? Are you trying to secure a "plum" residency and therefore want to get the highest grades possible for you, as well as make a good impression (by working overtime, by being superprepared for rounds, by volunteering for research projects) on your supervisors who will be writing your letters of reference? Or are you simply trying to pass; that is, you do not feel very confident and need to study hard to pass all your courses?

Whatever your reasons for studying, what is most important is that your partner is upset by the amount of time you devote to medical work. You must discuss this. Does your partner feel lonely, shoved aside, insignificant, hurt, or angry? Is your life out of balance? Is your partner bored with you, saying that you have become rather dull and no longer seem as interested in other things or things that you had in common?

What is the relationship of studying to your sexual life together? Do you frequently respond to sexual invitations with, "Sorry, I have to study." Do you no longer initiate sex like you used to? Do you yourself feel that your focus is principally school and that you have lost interest in making love? How worried are you about school and how you are doing? Are you thinking about school during lovemaking? Are you having trouble getting aroused—or having orgasms? Try to talk with your partner about this. My hunch is that you will feel better for it, just by getting things off your chest and having some support and understanding. It's been often said that physicians and medical students take themselves far too seriously. Your partner may know that and may help you lighten up, may get you laughing, and feeling relaxed again. The irony is clear: By divulging a concern that you are embarrassed about or all worked up about you will end up solving it—and having some fun in the bedroom! And you'll probably study much more productively and efficiently later

But studying can be a convenient excuse to avoid sexual intimacy. This can be both unconscious and conscious. In the former, you would have no idea at all that you are unhappy sexually and that you use studying as a cop-out. You may get hints of it in your dreams or through slips of the tongue or if you make sarcastic comments or if you have had too much to drink and say things that you deny the next day. If you are conscious of saying you have to study to avoid making love, you should try to be honest with yourself, examine it, and try to talk about it. The reasons for sexual avoidance are legion. Here are a few more common ones:

- Sex is physically painful.
- Sex together isn't fun anymore.
- You are not having orgasms anymore, and you have been faking them.
- You are furious at your partner for whatever reason, and because of anger you don't want to make love.
- You have lost respect for your partner and don't get aroused.

- You feel bullied into having sex by your partner, by his or her threats, manipulations, guilt trips, and physical aggression.

- You have lost interest in sex as a symptom of unrecognized depression in yourself.

- You are so panicky about your studies or life in general that sex is at the bottom of your priorities.

- You have been sexually abused or assaulted in the past and you feel confused sexually.

- You aren't happy in the relationship anymore and hence have lost interest in being intimate with your partner.

- You are confused about your sexual orientation but aren't ready to confront it yet.

Allan was a 25-year-old third-year medical student when he came to talk to me. His words were, "I think I know why I'm here. I'm living with my girlfriend, and I don't know what to do. I think it's over, but I don't know for sure, and the thought of breaking up really scares me." He continued: "Molly is a lovely woman. She's also in my class, but I think I got committed too young. She wants to get married, and I just want to run away. We met in first year, and it was magic. She's so beautiful, so smart, so athletic, so kind, so together, so perfect, but I've pulled away. Sex used to be terrific, transcending actually, but I shut down almost as soon as we set up house together last year. I got cold feet but couldn't bring myself to talk about it. The proverbial 'I didn't want to hurt her'—that's my excuse for lacking the guts and honesty to be straight with her. So we still have sex—occasionally— but I hate it, and it is sex, not lovemaking. I feel like a fraud. I am a fraud. I do it because I feel I should. But most of the time, I make excuses that I have to study, which is true. She's much smarter than me. But I use studying to keep the charade going. So I stay up late every night studying, and she goes to bed without me, or I tell her I prefer studying at the library or hanging out at the medical student center. And to really spill the beans, I'm really noticing other women these days. I want to start dating again."

My suggestion to Allan was very simple: He needed to have a heart-to-heart talk with Molly—which he did. She was sad, but not surprised. They made a decision to begin living apart at the end of the academic year. With the tension, misunderstanding, and pressure off, the two of them really enjoyed the rest of the term, both together and apart.

Why Do You Want to Talk All the Time?
Sex Is More Fun, Isn't It?

Guess who's making this statement? With very few exceptions, this is a male speaking. This tends to be a common gender difference in heterosexual couples. For women, talking achieves many purposes and is directly connected with feelings of closeness, trust, respect, and security. Talking includes the following: exchanging information in response to the question "How was your day?"; discussing something that one of you is struggling with; trying to solve a problem that you're having, a difference of opinion, a misunderstanding that has produced uncomfortable feelings in the two of you; chatting about family or friends; brainstorming about future plans together; gossiping about people at school or work; and so on. There is a feeling of connection during and after talking that makes lovemaking more possible and more enjoyable.

Men are not obsessed with sex, as this section title might suggest. But many men not only find having sex more enjoyable than (a lot of) talking but also find it a lot easier. And sometimes less time-consuming. And they would argue that they have a feeling of connection during and after lovemaking without having to do all of the talking beforehand.

Cary, a second-year medical student, and Annette, a writer, came to see me after giving birth to their stillborn son Brandon. Understandably, they were both intensely grieving this very painful and sad loss of their first child together. What was so troubling was that they could not agree on when and how much to speak about him. Annette couldn't talk enough about her feelings of love and sorrow, whereas Cary had really stopped wanting to talk about Brandon after his funeral. Now they were tense a lot of the time. And Annette had no interest in making love. Cary made this statement: "I've never felt very confident in how I use words to show my love for Annette. I try to show it when we make love. I feel even closer to her now, since Brandon's death, and I want to express it in bed. But she can't—yet. I miss him so much, and although he really never experienced life, I had a whole relationship with him that I had planned all through the pregnancy. There's an ache in my chest that won't go away, and it's worse when we don't make love." Looking at both of them, I asked,

"Have the two of you been able to talk about this." Annette replied, with tears in her eyes: "I had no idea that Cary felt all of this, about Brandon, about me, about our sexual relationship." They left the office holding hands. When they returned two weeks later, they both described talking a lot more—but also making love again as well.

A final word of caution: Never use sex as a panacea. Some couples say to themselves or each other, "Let's not talk, let's not fight, let's make love. Then we'll be back on track again." This may work occasionally or in the short run, but usually, one person feels worse afterward, more lonely and angry. This leads to erosion of joy and satisfaction, often to resentment, with the risk of complete sexual shutdown and divorce.

8 What About Extramarital Relationships?

Marriages and other committed intimate relationships are characterized by the expectation of fidelity throughout the life cycle. Although most married individuals take their vows very seriously, extramarital relationships for medical students and physicians are not uncommon. Nor are they uncommon in North American society. This does not lessen their sting, for any threat or assault to the sanctity or strength of the marital covenant almost always causes upset to marital function and integrity.

Extramarital Sex

Extramarital sex basically means that a married person has had sex on at least one occasion with someone outside the marriage. The two individuals may have had sex only once, with no expectation or interest in its continuing (the so-called one-night stand), or the two individuals may have had sex on several occasions. At one end of the continuum, sex may have occurred with little or no feeling for the person. At the other end of the continuum, there may have been an enormous amount of feeling and passion for each other. Although individuals who have had extramarital sex may defend themselves to their spouse that it was only sex and not a love relationship, this does not diminish the hurt for his or her partner. Put quite simply, the individual has broken the marital agreement, no matter how much he or she tries to explain it, make excuses for it, or play it down.

61

Extramarital Affair

An extramarital affair is a relationship that has developed between a married person and someone outside the marriage. It usually includes sex, but not always. Even when sex hasn't occurred, there is usually a recognition and disclosure that each of the parties makes of having developed affection and erotic feelings for each other along with either fear of or hope for consummation of those feelings at some future point. Extramarital affairs usually include loving and affectionate feelings for the person as well as a sense of longing. A person in an extramarital affair wishes to see the other individual again and sometimes, despite his or her best intentions, continues to do so. For many individuals, there is a very strong need to spend time together, and this may progress to an exciting or frightening feeling of being out of control. Most affairs involve a fair amount of inner conflict in one or both of the individuals as well as lots of deception. Whether or not a person feels guilty, and to what degree, varies from one individual to the next.

Not all individuals who are considering an affair or who are in the midst of one tell their spouses. Here are some of the times or situations in which an individual voluntarily reveals to his or her spouse the presence of a third party:

• When each member of the couple has vowed to tell each other absolutely everything, no matter how difficult or painful: These couples are actually in the minority. Although most couples believe they have this kind of openness with each other, when put to the test, it is usually a sham. One or both partners often hide an enormous amount from each other.

• When the person having the affair feels terribly guilty and cannot live with this feeling and the deceit any longer: When an extramarital affair progresses and results in a lot of lying and withholding of the truth, the individual's conscience gets the better of him or her, and the person needs the release that "fessing up" brings.

• When the person having the affair is reaching out to his or her spouse for support: The person is in need of help from his or her spouse and hopes, by disclosing what is going on, to better understand what's happening and that his or her spouse will assist in putting an end to the affair.

• When the person is leaving a marriage and he or she reveals the extramarital relationship because the intent is to continue with the other person: For the spouse who is left behind, this can be a nightmare because although the individual leaving explains the reason for the separation, it does not give the abandoned spouse any opportunity whatsoever to work on the marriage. And for the vast majority who did not suspect an affair or who did not see the separation coming, this can be absolutely overwhelming. The spouse left behind can literally feel "kicked in the stomach."

What about situations in which the individual does not voluntarily admit to the affair but is "found out." Here are some examples:

• When the spouse suspects that there is an affair, confronts his or her partner, and the person denies it; however, within a matter of hours or days, the individual admits that it is true: This is probably the most common type. Now that the affair is out in the open, the two individuals can begin to talk about it in earnest with a goal toward deciding what to do.

• When the person having the affair behaves in a haphazard or careless manner, making it appear that he or she wants or needs to be "found out." The person may be unavailable for hours at a time, may not go to classes or into work, may make secretive phone calls, especially late at night, may leave his or her Day-Timer or personal telephone book lying around, and so forth. These individuals often have a lot of difficulty owning up to their actions and have a history of not being very direct or truthful about what is going on with them. They tend to behave passively or passive-aggressively. Their behavior is usually very upsetting to those around them because they do not behave in a mature or responsible manner.

• When the individual has absolutely no desire, conscious or unconscious, to tell his or her spouse about the affair: The person is extremely careful about his or her actions and vigilantly leaves no clues. But because the person's behavior is different from before and he or she is tight-lipped or gone a lot, the person's spouse cannot help but become suspicious. He or she may follow the partner having an affair or think of other ways to catch him or her. In some situations, the spouse will hire a private investigator to confirm whether or not his or her partner is having an affair.

Why Do Extramarital Affairs Occur?

Individual Reasons

• *Immaturity.* These individuals have trouble honoring fidelity in marriage. Despite their chronological age, they may not have reached the stage of mature love. They tend to be self-centered individuals with poor control over their impulses. They have difficulty resisting the temptation to play out their sexual desires for other people.

• *Inner psychological conflict.* These people have problems with their self-esteem and do not feel very secure about themselves. In addition, they may not feel very confident sexually—or very confident at all. By getting love, attention, or sex from others, they feel affirmed and validated.

• *Disinhibition from alcohol or other drugs.* These individuals become sexually involved outside their marriages because they do not have the same inhibitions as they normally have when they are not drinking or using drugs. Examples are legion of individuals who would not have become sexually involved with each other if they were not drinking or using drugs.

• *Psychiatric illness, especially depression or bipolar illness.* Some individuals who are depressed are much more vulnerable to the interest or desires of someone in their environment who shows interest in them. In fact, because of the depression, their spouses may have withdrawn from them, which further compounds their sense of rejection or abandonment. Therefore, it is very exciting for them to be found attractive or intriguing by someone new. If someone has become hypomanic or manic, he or she may feel hypersexual in addition to having high energy and good spirits. That person is prone to extramarital affairs because he or she is behaving in both an extroverted manner and with poor judgment. That person does not assess people with the same degree of evaluation as he or she normally would, and because of this facilitated state, he or she takes chances and pushes normal boundaries.

• *Character deficiencies.* These individuals have a long-standing tendency not to be honest or trustworthy. This goes back to childhood or adolescence. Despite their protestations to the contrary, they are not really able to make a monogamous commitment to their spouse.

• *Sexual addiction.* These individuals are not very common, but their sexuality has a compulsive quality to it. They are driven to repeated sexual gratification from others, but the relief does not last very long. Soon it has to be satisfied again, either with the same person or with someone else. They frequently visit prostitutes, and some are also addicted to pornography.

• *Life cycle factor.* An example of this would be a person who has an affair around the age of 30. Sometimes these people are bored with their life, including their marriage, and they are drawn to the excitement that accompanies an affair.

• *Threats to one's job or career.* In this situation, the individual is vulnerable because his or her professional identity is threatened. If the person has lost a job, his or her self-worth is usually assaulted. The person may then be vulnerable to the support or soothing of someone outside his or her primary relationship who seems to care or who understands his or her predicament. This is usually somebody in the workplace.

Marital Reasons

Most people do not consciously and deliberately go out and start an affair. They may be vaguely aware of marital unhappiness or unrest, but many people in the midst of an affair are confused. Furthermore, many are surprised or shocked that this is their life. In other words, they had taken pride in their fidelity and thought that they would be the last person who would have an affair.

Some of the more common marital reasons for affairs are the following:

• *Boredom.* When people have been together a while, a state of sameness, predictability, or lack of stimulation may descend on them. People who are feeling somewhat disillusioned with their partners are at risk for and open to the excitement of an affair.

• *Loneliness.* Loneliness in marriage, unfortunately, is not uncommon. The two individuals are often together but do not feel connected or supported emotionally. Communication has either broken down or has never gone beyond being somewhat polite and superficial. Lonely people are sitting ducks for the attention or interest of others. Because they do not feel needed, loved, or adored by their spouses, they become very charged by the outside person. In fact, many of them resent their loneliness and feel used and abused by their spouses.

• *A spouse's preoccupation with work or business.* This dynamic is not uncommon in medical marriages wherein the medical student or physician partner is greatly preoccupied with studies or a career and his or her partner or spouse feels very left out. Many married people who are extremely busy have absolutely no insight into or understanding of how much they are neglecting their spouses. They find out very quickly, though, like being hit over the head with a baseball bat, when they learn that their spouse is having an affair.

• *When the spouse is ill.* When a spouse is chronically disabled with ongoing medical and/or psychiatric illnesses, the marriage can become extremely stressed. Spouses with disabling conditions are not able to function as well as able-bodied spouses. They may have difficulty meeting their partners' needs, doing things with their partners, holding up their responsibilities in the marriage, or being affectionate toward their partners. The healthy spouse can become resentful, fatigued, and quite isolated. He or she may long for the interest, affection, and companionship of someone else.

• *During a pregnancy or the postpartum stage.* When a man begins an affair during his wife's pregnancy or during the first postpartum year, it is often because of changed marital dynamics. In other words, he is not getting the same degree of attention and affection as he was getting before. Quite understandably, his wife is preoccupied with the pregnancy or extremely busy with a new baby. And his wife is usually exhausted.

Picking Up the Pieces After an Affair

If you are the one in your relationship who had the affair, you will feel a lot of loss that it is over. If you ended it, that will be a little easier because it was truly your decision. If the outside person ended it, you may feel abandoned on top of your feelings of grief. Or if your spouse insisted that you end it "or else," you may feel mad and resentful at him or her, even though you know that "you can't have your cake and eat it too."

You may have to mourn the affair once it's over, which means dealing with the following:

- Sorrow
- Longing and pining for the person
- Trouble concentrating and doing your studies, work, and so forth
- Preoccupation with the person, his or her appearance, memories together, shared intimacies, fantasies and dreams that the two of you might have had
- Inner emptiness, hollowness, numbness
- Crying spells that may wash over you like waves

Mourning is time limited, and if you do not contact each other, you will eventually feel better again. Time is the healer—and it takes time to mourn the person you adored or loved. Needless to say, your spouse needs to understand that you are mourning, that mourning accompanies lost love, and that it is very real. That said, this state is very frustrating for spouses because it can't pass fast enough for them. Your spouse wants you "back," wants to resume life with you, both the new you and the old you. It may take awhile for that enthusiasm to return when you both feel quite comfortable with your everyday rhythm together. And until a few weeks or months pass, most spouses are afraid, and rightly so, that you will go back on your word, that you will end the marriage to be with the other person.

Medical students, especially men but some women too, tend to be so busy with such demands on their time and attention, that they "compartmentalize" after they end an affair. In other words, they carry on quite successfully with studying, being on call, seeing patients, passing examinations, and applying for residency. It may appear that nothing happened or that they are not sad or regretful at all. Consciously, this is so because they really don't think about it much if at all. However, most are indeed grieving, but it is muted and done over time. Or it just sits somewhere—until the person has time and opportunity to process it at a later date.

Here is an example:

Zachary came to see me between first- and second-year medical school. He was doing summer research in neuroanatomy and neuropathology when he began to develop panic attacks and insomnia. He responded quickly to medication, but most important were the factors precipitating his symptoms. His father had died of a brain tumor five years earlier, so it made sense that attending autopsies and dissecting brains might be stressful for him. But he also told me that he had had an affair with another genetics grad student two years earlier when he was doing his master's degree before entering medical school. Although it went on for three months, he never told his wife, and he did not believe that she even suspected it. He ended the relationship because he couldn't live with himself any longer. He immediately pushed the experience away. "If thoughts of her entered my mind, I distracted myself right away with poems I had memorized or songs I had composed. Or I would think of my dad and how proud he'd be of me, applying to medical school and following in his footsteps. I just studied harder and harder. And it worked." Until his summer job, when he had less pressure. The panic symptoms were a message that he was bottled up and needed to release memories, thoughts, and feelings. Zachary benefited tremendously from talking about his father and how much he missed him, his guilt that he cheated on his wife, his guilt that his father would be disappointed in him too if he knew, and his guilt about the other woman and where her life was now and whether he had "screwed her up."

The First Year After the Affair Ends

If your husband or wife has had an affair, you will have many questions—and then more questions. If it is your husband who had the affair, don't be surprised if you get the feeling or message that he doesn't want to talk about it—and that you feel shut out and shut down. You want to talk. You need to talk. You are trying to understand it, to make some sense of how and why it happened, to get on track again with your spouse, to regain some marital security, to have your doubts relieved, to know your spouse more deeply and intimately, to know his or her conflicts and insecurities. And most of all, you want to make sure that it never happens again! Most individuals who have had an affair, once it is over, want to put it behind them, mourn as I described above, and carry on. They bristle when asked or forced to talk about it, usually because they feel ashamed and guilty and don't want to be reminded of it by talking about it. To quote one of many men, "My wife keeps bringing it up, over and over again. Why does she want to keep rubbing my face in it." Or, "She's going to make me pay for the rest of my life." Neither of these reasons are the real reasons; the real reasons are mentioned above—her need to understand and to connect again with her husband.

Most couples say that it takes at least a year for most of the wounds of an affair to heal and for trust to be more strongly restored. Rebuilding trust takes time, especially if or when the spouse who had the affair is out of town on trips or continues to work with or see the person with whom he or she was involved. There must be a simultaneous sense at home over the first year that the marriage bond feels stronger, that there is a coalition, that lovemaking is good or better than before, that communication is clean, direct, and honest. The first year after the affair can be rough, but it can also be beautifully close and touching, even magical—especially if the marriage had been strained or distant for months or years before the affair even began.

Warning Signals That You Are Vulnerable to an Affair

- You feel taken for granted at home. You don't feel that your spouse or partner really loves you, really wants you in his or her life.

- Your sexual relationship may be different—not as frequent, rote or mechanical, tense, less satisfying, less orgasmic. Or you may not be sexual at all anymore with your spouse or partner.

- You have been preoccupied with your relationship in a negative way—obsessing about it to yourself, feeling angry, ripped off, resentful.

- You begin to turn inward and pull away from your partner or spouse. You avoid talking with him or her. You don't look forward to coming home.

- You notice individuals more in your everyday world. They seem attractive to you, interesting. You want to spend time with them.

- You may begin to daydream (or dream) about someone else in your life who shows interest in you or who adores you.

- If or when you see this person, you feel excited, nervous, turned on. You would like to spend time with him or her.

- You actually plan or plot how you could be together with this person, ask him or her for coffee or a drink, opening up more about yourself than you have in a long time—or more than you ever have.

Let me end this chapter with two vignettes, very different, but with outcomes that address human frailty, strength, courage, and dignity.

Joseph called me on a Monday morning asking if he could see me as soon as possible. He was afraid: "I'm coming unglued." His voice was quivering, and he sounded very down. He told me that he was on call that evening and he didn't know if he should be working or not. I arranged to see him that afternoon. His story was that he had begun to spend "lots and lots" of time with Lori, an OB-GYN resident since starting his rotation at Women's Hospital. This began as coffee together, talks in the residents' lounge when they were on call together, and a few walks together on the university campus. Three days earlier, when he and Lori were postcall, they slept together back at her apartment. He immediately felt awful—and by his report, so did Lori. Joseph was married, and his wife was home full-time with their six-month daughter. Lori was married too; her husband was a resident in neurosurgery. My diagnosis was adjustment disorder with mixed anxiety and depressive symptoms. He was not clinically depressed, did not use or abuse substances, and his overall health was good. Joseph agreed to see me for a few visits until he felt better.

Here is what happened in treatment:

• I learned that Joseph had a huge amount on his plate and told him so. He was adjusting to being a new father, he was very busy on his clinical rotations, he was trying to get letters of reference for a particular program, so was trying especially hard to demonstrate his skills, he was working part-time as a bartender to make ends meet financially, and as a minority student, he felt that he had to be "flawless and not show any weakness, any cracks."

• I learned that Joseph's wife Mara was struggling too. She'd had a complicated pregnancy with bleeding in the third trimester, so she'd had to be on bed rest for weeks. Then she'd had a cesarean section, which went fine; however, she became moderately depressed and was on antidepressants. Although she was now well, that had been a tough time for the two of them. She'd had to stop breast-feeding, and that was hard for her. Her self-esteem was not good, and she had lost all interest in sex. Also, the baby had been sick a lot, which was a worry to both Mara and Joseph.

• Joseph was aware that his intense feelings for Lori were largely because things were not so good at home—that Mara was withdrawn a lot and sometimes irritable. She was busy with the baby, and he was on call or bartending a lot, so they were not "in sync" like before. He was kind of lonely, and Lori was fun and "very pretty."

• Sleeping with Lori was a wakeup call for Joseph. He had no intention of pursuing anything with her. He loved Mara and his daughter and had no thoughts whatsoever of breaking up the family or of "doing anything stupid— like thinking I can have both."

• I had three sessions with Joseph and Mara together to address some of the adjustment issues they were coping with as a young family of three. These visits went very well; their marriage was a strong one with lots of love, maturity, and willingness to compromise. They did well.

* * *

Donald and Michelle gave this as their chief complaint: "We really love each other, but we got problems—big time." And indeed they did. Each of them was intimately involved with someone else. Donald was an attorney, and he had been seeing an actress for a few months. Michelle was an attorney as well, but she was now a first-year medical student. She had become very close with a man in her class and was spending "lots of time with him." Both Donald and Michelle were aboveboard with each other—and with the individuals they were seeing. Their questions to me were these: "Are we fooling ourselves to think we love each other or what? If we do, why are we pushing things? Are we both two grown-up kids who can't just accept one partner? We need to sort this out." I agreed.

Donald and Michelle met in law school and began living together within a few weeks. They were dazzled by each other. They were both very attractive, smart, dynamic, elite athletes, politically savvy, and well traveled. They also came from similar backgrounds— moneyed families but homes that were very chaotic and insecure with physical and sexual abuse, several divorces, alcoholism, suicide, and white-collar crime. They had been living together for six years when I met them, with no intention of marrying—ever. They thought marriage was an anachronism—legally and spiritually confining—and certainly not for them. However, they felt married, until their outside relationships began. From what I could tell, they each drifted into these relationships—partly out of excitement (they each admitted that they liked new people who were "different") and partly out of boredom with each other. And because they saw themselves as progressive liberals, morally they had no problem with outside partners. However, when pressed, they each admitted to me privately in individual visits that they felt threatened by these third and fourth parties—and that they were competing and partly trying to make each other jealous and to "test" the other's commitment.

Here is what I did:

• I told them both that I could not help them as a couple as long as they had relationships going on elsewhere and to rethink if they really wanted to work on their relationship or not. I asked them to go away and think about that. I did not expect to hear from them again, but they called in about a month. They had each stopped seeing the people they were involved with.

• We began to meet weekly, but I was tentative and low-key with them because I knew that they were trying to get over their girlfriend and boyfriend. I was struck by how open they were with each other about these other individuals and the sadness and guilt that they felt about "using" other people. This process seemed to bring them closer.

• I also began to more deeply understand how much Michelle and Donald were "soulmates." Neither of them had ever really opened up to others like they had with each other—probably because their backgrounds were so painful and so unrelenting in repeated losses that they didn't trust people to understand or to accept them. They were survivors who found solace in each other.

• I told them that I thought their "affairs" were partly explained by life cycle (Michelle was 30 and Donald was 31) and by acting out against each other. That in addition to being lovers and partners, they were each somewhat parental with the other. This was because neither of them really had a stable or consistent mother or father while growing up (they were sent away to boarding schools, and their parents kept divorcing, remarrying, and redivorcing or were living abroad and not in close communication). This seemed to make sense to them, because indeed they did tend to parent the other in lots of ways—mainly good ways, caretaking ways, more than controlling ways.

• They worked hard at my suggestions to them about wholesome communication in marriage and some homework exercises that I gave them, which they seemed to enjoy. The three of us were aware that they really didn't grow up with mutually respectful adult-to-adult role models, so this was very foreign to them.

• And then Michelle became pregnant. After the initial shock, they were thrilled. They surprised each other because their mantra together had always been "no kids." And they also surprised each other by deciding to get married!

• My last visit was with the three of them (they had a beautiful baby boy they called Leo) and things were going well. Michelle was on maternity leave from medical school, and Donald had reduced his trial work so that they would have more time together as a family.

9 Maybe We Should Just Break Up

Stop Threatening Me!

The statement "Maybe we should just break up" can't help but be perceived as threatening—even if you don't mean to be threatening in intent or tone. Here are several possible statements, that may or may not be stated aloud, that could precede "Maybe we should just break up."

- You put me down so much. Maybe . . .
- You're always angry at me. Maybe . . .
- So you're disappointed in me again, are you? Maybe . . .
- You seem interested in other guys (or women). Maybe . . .
- I can't stand your bitching at me all the time. Maybe . . .
- Look, this relationship is hopeless. We're both miserable. Maybe . . .
- I really don't think that healthy relationships should be this awful. Maybe . . .
- I want out. Stop laying guilt trips on me. Maybe . . .
- (and rarely uttered aloud) I don't love you anymore. Maybe . . .

All of these statements say that something has changed—that the two of you are not as happy. Or certainly, one of you isn't. Other emotions? Confusion, a sense of loss of what once was, sadness, resentment, frustration, and disillusionment, or maybe you feel trapped. It is hard to tell whether or not this is just a bad spell in a relationship and you should just "batten down the hatches" or if this really is the beginning of the end. What follows is an example of each:

Chuck, a first-year medical student, and Carla, a flight attendant, came with this as a chief complaint, spoken by Chuck but echoed by Carla: "We came today because we don't know whether we need therapy to try to improve things or whether we should just cut our losses, shake hands, and go our separate ways." I quickly learned by some examples that they each gave that their communication was the pits, that they really couldn't discuss the weather without fighting. In fact, they bickered most of the visit and kept interrupting each other when one was trying to tell a story about their problem. They each remembered different details. Chuck was especially fed up and demoralized; in fact, he referred to breaking up at least three times in the one-hour visit. Carla tended to taunt him when he spoke like that, using what I thought was the age-old mechanism of the best defense is an offense. My intuitive sense was that these two had a viable relationship. I told them that and that I thought a few visits together would be helpful. I also told them that if I was wrong, we would know that in a few visits, too.

Here is what seemed to help:

• I told Chuck that he had to try to stop his "Maybe we should just break up" statements, and when he did forget and didn't realize it, Carla should say something like, "There you go again, pulling the plug" rather than going off like a torpedo with comments such as "There's the door. Get the f . . . k out right now!"

• I suggested to Chuck that he try to examine what he's feeling when he's about to make one of his breakup statements—and to speak the feeling. Pretty soon, he was able to say things such as, "I'm getting really angry again about the way we can't talk about anything," or "Carla, I'm feeling hopeless again, please let me finish this story; then you respond," or "This conversation is making me really upset. When you tell me yet again that I should be studying, I feel ashamed and guilty."

• Carla was delighted that Chuck was talking about his feelings. I did, however, ask her to try to be patient when and if he needed some alone time to process what he was feeling. She agreed to work on that.

• Through talking about their backgrounds and families together, they were able to see how they had developed this dynamic with each other. Chuck's parents fought constantly for most of his childhood before they divorced when he was a teenager. He recalled frequent fantasies of running away to a peaceful home somewhere where he could be alone—hence, his adult response, in the face of arguing or misunderstandings: "Maybe we should just break up." Carla had tremendous separation anxiety. Her mother, a single parent, drank a lot and also got depressed. She threatened suicide when she was down or was fed up with Carla and her younger brothers. Carla also had had a previous boyfriend who not only was married while he was seeing her but who also had another girlfriend besides Carla. Hence, her insecurity came out in the form of rage when Chuck referred to breaking up.

• Finally, I suggested that the two of them look very carefully at their busy lives, get a huge calendar and two pocket Day-Timers and slot in time as soon as Carla received her flying schedule. She flew overseas so was away for blocks of time but was also off for several days in a row. And Chuck worked part-time as a nurse, so he had different shifts, too, that needed to be entered onto the schedule. I explained that at least part of their communication trouble was that they needed to recognize that their interdependence was different from couples who saw each other daily, that they frequently had to shift from "alone" mode to "together" mode, and that this is a dance. They just establish a rhythm, and the music is over—when Carla had to leave to go overseas or Chuck was on evening shift and they didn't see each other for several days.

The situation and outcome were very different for this next couple:

Marcus was a final-year medical student, and his wife Anne was home full-time as a mother to their one-year-old son. They both complained that things were grim, that they were going through the motions of being a couple, and that they were concerned about the effects their tension and bickering had on William, their son. Anne wanted to discuss separation. She said that she didn't love Marcus anymore, but they couldn't discuss this on their own because Marcus believed that they should get help and stay together for William—and because, although he was no longer a practicing Catholic, he didn't believe in divorce. In his mind, "Kids from broken homes were all screwed up." Marcus also argued that Anne was angry at him because he had a three-week affair with one of his classmates when Anne was pregnant and that she was trying to punish him by breaking up the marriage. Anne responded that she wasn't angry at him; she was disgusted—and that that was only the tip of the iceberg, that there were all kinds of ways in which she felt she made a mistake getting involved with a man "who cares about absolutely no one except himself—and maybe William." Here is a summary of my treatment with them:

- I met with each of them alone (which is my usual practice). I detected some ambivalence on Anne's part—that she was very hurt and furious at Marcus for many things but that she still did love him in some ways—and she did have mixed feelings about the impact of divorce on William and his future development. I found Marcus quite immature and not really ready for the responsibilities of marriage and fatherhood. He admitted that he was very attracted to other women and had viewed Anne as a mother figure even before they got married. "It's hard to get turned on by someone who's always right— and so sensible—but I try." He thought he'd better stay married, or "My father will kill me. He's on faculty here at the medical school, and like Anne, he always does the right thing. He wouldn't leave my mother even though they have been miserable for years."

- I told them both that we should "try" marital therapy. We spent the first few visits talking about difficult subjects—their on-again, off-again courtship; Anne's miscarriage of an earlier pregnancy; Marcus's having to repeat a year of medical school; Anne's being overweight; and Marcus's affair. At first, it seemed that uncovering and airing these hurts and losses in a supportive and safe atmosphere was helping—that is, that they understood each other better and that there was some forgiveness on both of their parts. However, this didn't continue. They began to avoid setting aside any time at home to talk between sessions and began to spend more time talking with their individual friends. They no longer had any couple friends, which is always a bad sign.

- When they each missed coming to a joint visit and just the other came, I realized that there was a growing sense that this wasn't working—that they were increasingly sealed off from each other. Both brought up separation now.

- We then moved into separation therapy over the next few visits. They were each relieved yet sad and anxious, but now they were very cordial together and had many good times when the three of them did things as a family. They negotiated on a point when Marcus would move out and talked easily about visitation, finances, dividing up their possessions, and other housekeeping matters.

To his surprise, Marcus found his father and mother very understanding about the separation. Anne's parents were as well. I saw them together for a few visits after they separated, over the first year, and except for a bit of a setback when each of them began to date other partners, everything went quite smoothly.

In this chapter, I have attempted to illustrate that a feeling of "maybe we should just break up" can mean different things. It may be the most logical and rational outcome of trying your best, and therefore a decision to go your separate ways will be both appropriate and healthy. However, a feeling of "maybe we should just break up" can also be a response to overwhelming frustration, exhaustion, and ennui. Breaking up feels like it would be a relief, and perhaps it would be—in the short term. When in doubt, go see someone and get a professional opinion on the best course to take.

10

I Wish I Knew Whether This Was Normal or Not

Everyone Else Seems So Happy!

"All our friends are so happy" were the words of Jenn, a stockbroker married to Jeff, a third-year medical student. At least that was how Jeff quoted Jenn when he came to see me on his own. He was really worried that Jenn was so unhappy being married to him, that she wasn't sure she wanted to stay with someone who was going to be a doctor. She complained that he was not any fun, that he was too serious, that he was "obsessed with medicine," that he had nothing else to talk about, and that his friends in medicine were all like him "kind of arrogant—and kind of uptight." Jeff told me that he really loved Jenn and that he had to agree with her in lots of ways—that life together wasn't really much fun and that she was a little disappointed with him. He seemed worried and down. I thought they could benefit from a few couples visits and told him that. He didn't think that Jenn would come in. He hadn't told her that he had made an appointment with me. He thought that she would "tease" him as being "weak" or respond with "Yes, you really do need professional help; you're too rigid, too hung up."

To Jeff's surprise, Jenn was more than willing to come in. She was thrilled, actually, that he cared enough about the two of them to go see someone. I saw her alone. Her story was somewhat different from Jeff's. Yes, she was unhappy, but not hopeless. She really loved him but did feel that he and his classmates took themselves far too seriously, that they needed to enjoy life more. She was very friendly, outgoing, and hardworking herself but good at leaving her work at work and pursuing her athletic interests and other hobbies. She had an engaging sense of humor, and I thought that their relationship was very complementary. She admitted that Jeff did help to keep her on track at times and that she made him laugh at himself, occasionally, but not often enough.

I scheduled a few visits for the two of them together. And we talked about "Is this normal or not?" I reassured them that lots of male physician marriages were like theirs and that there was lots of room for the two of them to have more happiness together. I also told Jeff that he would be able to relax more as he progressed through medical school and residency, that he shouldn't study as much as he was, that he had to strive for balance, that he would never "know it all," and that he was fortunate to have a partner like Jenn who was so candid with him and who wanted the best possible relationship they could have together. I told Jenn that her world of the stock exchange was very different from Jeff's and that that was good—and not to despair that they had nothing in common. In fact, on their own, they decided to spend a half-day visiting each other's workplace so they could each "be a fly on the wall" and get a sense of their different worlds.

And I mentioned to them, which they inherently knew, that their perception of their friends all being so happy, was no more than perception. That they too may be struggling and having their own particular challenges.

*   *   *

"Compared with my parents, our relationship is like heaven!"
"Compared with my parents, our relationship is like hell!"
"Stop comparing us with other couples!"

These statements aren't uncommon when one member of a couple is feeling threatened or defensive about their relationship and is trying to respond to a partner who is complaining about the marriage, who wants to do something about it, who is unhappy with the status quo, who doesn't want to be compared with other couples, who simply wants things to be better. A partner who perhaps has a belief or principle that "I am not a complacent person. I am not going to go through life with a relationship that is just so so. I want a relationship that is alive, creative, dynamic, fun, and forever evolving. I refuse to accept this as the best that I, that we, can achieve."

Here are some other questions that individuals in intimate relationships may ask themselves or each other:

• *Should a relationship be this challenging?* All relationships have challenges—some more than others and some at different times and stages of a relationship. It's very hard to know how one's relationship compares with others. And as much as one shouldn't compare, there is a natural tendency to do that. It probably represents an effort to understand, to want to reassure oneself and each other, or perhaps it's an effort not to deal with a problem that is staring you in the face. It may be a way of minimizing things—that is, "Our relationship is not that bad, is it?"

• *What are the norms?* There is no easy answer to this question. How normal is it to argue, to fight, to have days of not speaking, to have your sex life wane, to have fantasies of other partners, to want to separate? Most experts would say that all of the above are quite normal. And lots of couples who have been together for a long time would probably agree. However, lots of divorced individuals would say they experienced all of the above and didn't make it. The key is degree and duration. Ominous signs are big arguments or arguments over "everything" or unrelenting arguments day after day after day; fighting that gets mean with lots of name-calling, abusive language, threats, swearing, and physical or sexual violence; days of not speaking become weeks; infrequent sex or no sex at all or the opposite, frequent sex but without feeling or meaning; fantasies of other partners turn into reality and you start an affair; lots of thoughts of going your separate way, thoughts that aren't frightening anymore, thoughts that give you lots of relief.

• *I had no idea that relationships take this much work!* Again, this is highly subjective. All relationships require some work, some effort. But given your personality and whether you have more than a few conflicts, your relationship may take more work. If you got committed or married quite young, you may not have the maturity to flow with the good and the bad of a relationship. If your self-esteem isn't very good, you may not take constructive criticism very well from your partner; you see any criticism as an attack, and you attack back very defensively or you are easily wounded and become silent for hours or days. If your parents did not really model for you how to talk with respect and honor to a loved one, you may find this difficult. You will need some education and practice. If you were abused as a child, you may become quite fearful, panicky, phobic, or paralyzed in the face of anger or heated discussions. Therefore, it is hard for you and your partner to really tackle and overcome your differences with each other. If your home life growing up was suppressed or repressed and nobody really spoke their true feelings (i.e., the atmosphere was sanitized, always pleasant but somehow not real), then any strong emotion or confrontation will feel very foreign to you. You will need assistance in how to identify your inner feelings and how to respond with honesty to your partner.

• *Why aren't we as happy as we were in the early weeks of meeting each other, dating, and getting to know each other?* Ah, wouldn't everyone like to return to that phase of a relationship, the phase of discovery and anticipation of all good things. You're probably longing for that and feeling sad that you don't have it. I suggest reframing the question from such a passive lament to a proactive quest: "Let's try to find each other again. Let's try to create a new version of our early days and weeks together. I believe in us. I think we can rediscover each other."

• *I'm so confused.* I really still love you, I think, but the thought of my own place is really appealing—being on my own, with no one to have to answer to, to have to support, to have to cook for, clean up for. Have I gotten tied down too young? But you don't seem to feel the same way as me. You seem to like being married. And that makes me feel very guilty—and like I've failed. These are hard questions to have to ask oneself or to discuss with each other. But if you're asking them, you need to discuss them with each other.

Suggestions

• You need a "reality check." Talk to a friend about how you are feeling. If your friend is someone who has a lot, or at least some, experience with relationships, he or she may be able to give you a perspective on the way you are feeling, the way you are viewing your relationship. This kind of talk could be very reassuring. Your friend may see your state as purely situational, as a phase, or as temporary. In fact, a friend may give you some good advice and guide you and support you through this very difficult time.

• If you have discussed the way that you are each feeling and are friendly with a couple whom you really respect as good listeners and who like both of you and who have each of your best interests at heart, speak to them about what you are experiencing. They may have experienced some or all very similar feelings or conflicts themselves—and have resolved them. They may have some good counsel to give. If your relationship with one or both sets of your parents is good, why not speak to them about your marriage? They too may have insights into each of you that they have never spoken about, and of course, having been at your stage of a relationship themselves before, they may have some words of wisdom for the two of you. And they may appreciate your reaching out to them and respecting their judgment and life experience.

• Consider a visit or two with a couples therapist. This individual will certainly be able to give you a "diagnostic impression" of what is going on from his or her perspective. This should be very helpful. And it may give each of you something concrete, some explanation for the way you are feeling and why—and what can be done about it. This may involve more couples work, individual treatment for one or both of you, some recommended reading material, some homework, perhaps a couples group, or a marital enrichment weekend. There are lots of possibilities.

11 I Worry About Our Kids

"We're both students, and we work and study so hard that I'm afraid that our kids will grow up thinking my mom is their mom. I just wish that we, each of us, had more time with them."

Yours is a very common, and very understandable, concern. It's fine—and healthy—to have regrets and to talk with each other about them; however, it isn't fine to berate yourself. What is key is to build on what you do have and make the best of your situation. Your decision to become a physician is probably as central in your life as being a mother or father. Here are some suggestions that might make you feel better.

Map out as best you can what your week looks like in terms of hours spent at home, at school, at the hospital, and outside the home for other reasons. Protecting a few extra minutes or hours at the beginning of the day, end of the day, or weekends to spend with your child(ren) will ease your conscience and bring satisfaction. Do this exercise over a week's or month's time as well. This will help you to plan for those times of the month when there are statutory holidays, vacation, spring break, and so forth. Knowing that you have a week off in a few weeks helps you to feel less guilty if you are on a particularly demanding service or have examinations coming and you haven't had as much time with your family as you would like. Use the telephone liberally and often to snatch a few minutes conversation with your son or daughter—or to reinforce parenting matters when you are not able to be at home ("Did you do your math homework? Make sure you brush your teeth? I'll read you a longer story tomorrow night when I'm home").

If you are generally pleased with your child care arrangement and feel that your child is in good hands and is safe, that will free you up to focus on your studies and/or medical work. The opposite is true in spades. It is impossible to ignore those intrusive or panicky thoughts that flood your mind in the middle of a lecture or clinic if you are worried about the care your child is getting. Pay attention to these thoughts—and act! It is the rare mother who is irrationally anxious about her loved ones at home. Don't let your husband shame or manipulate you into feeling that you are "making a mountain out of a molehill." If your mother or mother-in-law is your caretaker, discuss your concerns. You will feel better having your fears allayed. If you need to change day care settings or get a different nanny or babysitter, do it. You have to feel that your kids are getting the best care they can get, short of having you do it.

Try to remember that your medical school years are finite—that this is a critical but time-limited period in your life. Although it corresponds with critical developmental years of your child, with the right attitude, you can put yourself at ease and make the best of your situation. Try to remember that even if you were able to be home full-time with your son or daughter, there is no way of knowing whether that would be better for your child or not. Even full-time mothers have conflicting interests and time demands. Try to see that, for you, being fulfilled with your career plans makes you a better and happier mother.

Much of what I have said above applies to your husband as well. Accept that you won't be able to study as much as a classmate with no responsibilities to a spouse or child. Do not use your medical career, and its demands, as an excuse. Your modus operandi should be this: I want to be the best medical student, spouse, and parent that I can be, given my circumstances. All three should have equal valence.

With both of you being medical students and parents, your financial resources are probably spare. Make sure that you do try to budget a few dollars each month for the two of you to go out on a date, to have some alone time as a couple outside your home. Once every two weeks is minimal. Use the money for the babysitter and simply go for a walk or sit on a park bench and talk for a couple of hours if money is especially tight.

* * *

"You're a medical student; I'm working full time. I wish that one of us could be a stay-at-home parent."

Your situation is similar to the above. I imagine that you have brainstormed to the best of your abilities to see if any other arrangement would work. One of you has to work for all of you to live. And work may also be essential for your psychological well-being. Or it may be part of your career trajectory; if you stop work, you will not be able to continue in your field of training and expertise. Here are some additional suggestions.

Make sure that you are not working at your job any harder than you need to. Don't take on any unpaid committee or volunteer work unless you have discussed that at home and have worked out a compromise that you are both happy with. Intimate, hands-on contact with your child is much more important than work-related commitments—and a much more rewarding investment!

Is there any way to maximize your earning potential with fewer hours at work? Are you making as much money as you should be, given your talent and expertise? Could you find work that paid the same but demanded fewer hours so that you could be at home more and not have to rely as much on paid help for your child? Is there any way you can combine part-time work outside the home with part-time work in the home?

(To the medical student spouse) Is there any way that you can be at home more hours per week without compromising your studies and responsibilities? Do you have skills or previous work experience that allow you to work part-time to contribute to the running of the house, thereby freeing up your working spouse a bit from bearing full financial responsibility? Examples include typing of manuscripts and other at-home transcription work, nursing a few shifts each month, using your pharmacy degree to work in a drugstore part time, driving a taxicab, tutoring, giving music lessons, teaching racket sports, being a life guard, gardening, working in the university library, and assisting professors with research or laboratory experiments.

Make sure that you talk frequently with each other about fairness in terms of how you divide up your child care responsibilities and domestic chores. I see many medical student couples each year wherein one or both of the spouses feels shortchanged, bitter, and resentful that they are doing more than their share. This is sometimes the medical student, sometimes his or her working spouse. Your starting point should be that at the end of the day—say, 5 or 6 p.m. when you arrive home—you are both tired, and there must be an equitable distribution of work in the home from that point on and on the weekends. Being a medical student who has to study must never be used as a cop-out to avoid work and child care responsibilities in the home. Similarly, working outside the home all day should not be seen as "harder work" than being a medical student sitting in class all day or attending clinics and rounds.

* * *

"I don't think that this is a healthy way for kids to grow up—with this tension, with us fighting all the time."

I agree! I'm glad that at least one of you, and maybe both of you, are concerned. Here are some thoughts on how to make it better.

What do you mean by "tension"? Something you can feel in the air when you are together? Not speaking to each other? Speaking to each other in a defensive, clipped, sharp, or sarcastic tone? Something you feel in your body—a knot in your stomach, migraine or tension headaches? Try to tease this out with each other.

What do you mean when you say you are "fighting all the time"? Arguing? Bickering? Calling each other names? Threatening each other? Blaming each other? Hitting each other? Try to discuss this. Does your spouse agree? How would he or she describe what you are articulating?

Each of you should ask yourself in a reflective way: "Why is this happening?" Why the tension, the fighting? Look inward to try to identify what and how much you personally are bringing to the table. Examples might be the following:

"I'm worried about exams. I think I might fail."

"I'm worried about money. How are we going to be able to get the car fixed and still pay the rent this month?"

"I'm worried about my health. Am I depressed?"

"Do I have cancer?"

"I'm tired of being picked on. I'm not taking it anymore. I'm on the defensive constantly now because I'm fed up."

"I'm not sure if I want to be married anymore. I'm thinking about separation a lot these days. I just need some alone time."

"I'm exhausted. My nerves are shot. I feel like I'm premenstrual all month long now."

"I'm on edge night and day. I feel like I want to rip somebody's face off. I feel like I'm premenstrual—and I'm a man!"

"Since my father committed suicide last fall, I'm not the same as I used to be."

"I love our kids—more than you could ever know—but I resent them, too. If it weren't for them, I'd be gone gone gone from this lousy marriage."

Set aside some time to try to talk to each other about what you have learned by looking inward, what you have identified that might be contributing to the

mood at home. Listen carefully to each other. It should help to hear your partner speak about his or her contribution to the difficulty at home. Acknowledge
this and be supportive. Even if you believe that the way you feel is a direct result of the way you perceive your spouse to be, you should be able to express
this without attacking or blaming or threatening. Compare these two statements, both expressing the same sentiment but with different emphasis:

> "I know I've turned into a witch, but I find you so tense these days, with exams ap-
> proaching, and I feel so picked on by you that I go off like a rocket the minute
> you open your mouth. My self-esteem at the moment is very shaky, so I'm
> pretty defensive."

> "You're impossible to live with. You yell constantly. I dread seeing you at the end of
> the day because you're always in a rotten mood. You're screwing up Andrea
> with all of your putdowns. I think you need psychiatric help."

If you are successful at this, you may be able to work out many of your misunderstandings on your own as a couple. What is important is that you stop analyzing your partner and analyze yourself—not an easy exercise. Most people
in a marriage have a lot more insight into their spouse's shortcomings than their
own. This is one of the reasons that spouses get defensive and feel blamed by
the other—and that communication breaks down.

If the above does not seem to work or help, get some marital therapy. A
trained, objective, and neutral professional will be able to help sort out what is
happening and make suggestions to the two of you to make the atmosphere at
home happier, more functional, and not traumatic for your children.

*   *   *

She says, "You're always studying or you're at the hospital. I understand because I'm an adult. But poor Joshua doesn't even realize that
he has a father."

He says, "Thanks for the guilt trip." (Unspoken: "as if I didn't feel
shitty enough already. You really know how to rub my nose in it,
don't you?")

The above exchange is not uncommon in busy medical student marriages
with children. Obviously, this woman is very worried about her son's relationship with his father. She wants it to be better. She wants her son to have more
time with his dad. She is his mouthpiece, which may be appropriate because he

time with his dad. She is his mouthpiece, which may be appropriate because he is too young to say it or perhaps he has told her but not his father how much he would like more time with his daddy. She may also be identifying with Joshua and projecting this outward; that is, she recalls her own relationship with her father at this age and if it was particularly good, she would like to re-create that for Joshua. If, on the other hand, she felt deprived of her dad's time and companionship, she may want to spare her son that aching or longing and is prepared to fight to ensure that her son has a better relationship with his father than she herself had. Furthermore, as a contemporary and/or progressive parent, she realizes that kids thrive better when they have the love, play, discipline, and time of *both* parents, so she wants that. And because Joshua is a boy, she especially wants her son to have the identification figure and role model of an involved father. Here are my suggestions toward perhaps achieving that.

Delete the above statement to your husband. How about something like this? "Can I talk to you about your relationship with Joshua? As you know, you don't get a lot of time with him because you have to study a lot or be at the hospital until late. Do you think there's any way you could go in late some days and have breakfast with him or come home for an hour at noon, or get home a bit earlier to play with him or read him his bedtime story?" This is invitational, it's clear, and it gives options.

Perhaps your husband responds with something like this: "I agree. I've been worried about my relationship with him. He's growing so fast. I should be able to get home for lunch on Tuesdays and Thursdays before clinic."

What if your husband says this? "What're you getting at? I get lots of time with Joshua. He knows how busy I am. He gets a hell of a lot more time with me than I ever got with my dad at his age. And I do more with him than Jim (a classmate) and his son." I recommend your responding with something like, "I agree that you two have a good relationship. I just think it could be a bit better. I know how busy you are, but could you just think a bit about my suggestions? I don't think boys can ever get too much time with their dads."

This example could lead to a very fruitful talk about competing commitments. Your husband may welcome the opportunity to talk about how tough it is to be a good student doctor, husband, and father—and that he feels kind of guilty that he doesn't have more time with Joshua or jealous of your relationship with him or resentful that his schedule is so tightly packed. It will feel good just to identify and ventilate these feelings.

Make sure that you clarify that it is just Joshua you are concerned about. Is it possible that you feel deprived of time with your busy husband yourself? If so, that is a whole other area for the two of you to talk about.

Finally, a good-faith talk like this will give the two of you a chance to brainstorm creative ways, in addition to your suggestions above, for Joshua and his dad to have more one-to-one time together.

* * *

"I think you might have a postpartum depression. I just learned about that in Psych. Why? Because you're always tired, and you're so busy with the baby that you're always yelling at little Carlos. Poor kid. I feel sorry for him. It's a wonder he has any self-esteem anymore the way you treat him."

Talk about laying guilt trips! Obviously, this concern needs to be talked about but leave out the part about Carlos's self-esteem—and the *always* in the sentence. How about this? "Another symptom you might have is irritability. I find you kind of touchy with me and kind of short with Carlos. I know he's in the terrible twos but . . ." Hopefully, your wife will respond better with this approach. Talking about depression isn't easy. What is pivotal is that your wife not feel attacked, criticized, or blamed. In fact, she might be relieved that you have noticed that she's out of sorts—and that you care. If she has more symptoms of depression and they have been going on more than two weeks, she should talk to her primary care physician about the way she's feeling. And if at all possible, you should go with her on that visit.

* * *

"We should have waited to have kids—until I was out of training."

This statement probably means nothing more than you're having a bad day or going through a rough patch of too much on your plate. Try to remember the following:

- All parents have regrets or concerns at times about the timing of their kids.

- Sure, having kids is easier at certain times of one's life than others, but we don't always have that kind of control or personal choice of when we have kids—their spacing or even how many. If your children are planned, you probably gave a lot of thought to having kids during training as opposed to waiting.

Try to remember your reasons then and stop berating yourself. If your children are (or one of your children is) unplanned, for whatever reason(s), that's life. Those things happen. And those things happen to smart people like you and your spouse.

• I make the above statements because each year I see medical students or residents who find themselves with an unplanned pregnancy. They tend to be hard on themselves. They feel that because of good awareness about family planning, they should not be in this situation. Once again, these things happen. And they happen to smart people.

• The two of you should talk about the issue of having children and its implications for your lives. Does having kids affect your options? Your budget? Your debt load? Your housing? Which residency you choose? Your flexibility regarding that residency? The employment and/or career path of your spouse? The role dynamics of your marriage? Have you gone from a two-earner marriage to a single-earner relationship? Has the balance of power shifted? Does one of you feel that you are doing more than your share of the domestic work? Do you feel that your marriage is getting short shrift because of kids—that is, that the two of you don't get much time alone as a couple and you resent that, thinking that if you had waited a few years to have kids you wouldn't have to share each other as much as you do now?

* * *

"I wish that our parents didn't live so far away. Our kids don't know their grandparents. Plus, it would be nice to get away together for a weekend and have them baby-sit."

This is a common reality for many couples today—the so-called nuclear family residing some distance from their extended family. Here are some thoughts.

Carefully review your budget with the goal of a weekend away sometime in the next few months. Is it possible that your sitter or nanny can be available? At what cost? If you have friends who also have a child or children, would they be interested in an exchange? That is, you look after their kids for a quick get away and they reciprocate another time. Any possibility of a parent coming for a short visit to see all of you who also is interested and willing to look after the kids for a couple of days?

Regarding your kids having a relationship with their grandparents, this may get easier when you have more disposable income after medical school that allows for a summer or holiday visit to your respective families. This is not the same as living in the same community as your parents, but it is better than no relationship at all. And you may be able to plan your professional future in a way that allows you, in a few years, to practice where your family or families live—or nearby.

12 Intermarriages Can Be Tough!

Given the cultural mosaic of our medical schools, a number of you may be dating someone or be involved in an intimate relationship with someone who is of a different race, religion, or ethnic group from yourself. For most of you, this is either a nonissue or completely eclipsed by the love that you feel for each other. In other words, you are blind to the differences in your families of origin, cultural values, skin color, food preferences and idiosyncrasies, holidays, and where you worship. For some of you, it is very different; you initially were or now are, drawn to the other's customs, family members, or faith, and these stand out as intriguing and binding dynamics that give your relationship a secure foundation. If you were somewhat rudderless before you met, you now have ballast with your partner. Whatever the specifics, most people in interfaith, interethnic, or interracial relationships, describe excitement, wonder, challenge, and enrichment, due to the fascinating blend of their backgrounds, customs, and values.

Let me speak, however, about some of the challenges and problems that are not uncommon and that have formed the focus of my therapy with medical student couples in my practice. Remember that lots of these are temporary and transitory. That is, they are all part of "the getting to know each other" or "disillusionment" phase of a relationship that occurs after a few months of dating, living together, or marriage. It hits you in the face or in the gut—the inner sense of "we are really very different" or the statement "I had no idea that you felt so strongly about this." It can be scary, and you may have a lot of feelings of regret that you got involved in the first place, or you may be upset with yourself that you didn't see this or that—or minimized it. You may also feel duped—that your partner wasn't clear or honest with you about his or her adherence to religious or family tenets or rules.

Have You Underestimated Your Differences?

How do you know this? Acknowledge that the glow of the early weeks or months of your courtship has dimmed a little and you are much more familiar and analytical with each other. You both may be examining each other as someone to whom you are making a commitment—or to whom you already have made a commitment. The differences you noticed at the beginning or even well into the early phases of your relationship did not seem insurmountable. Now they do. Try to remember that you may be going through a rough patch—that is, a stressful time during which your very different coping styles come to the fore. If there is quite a cultural divide, this may feel kind of lonely—and frightening. What started out as a stressor totally unrelated to your "intermarriage" or "interrelationship" now has you fighting about it! Here is an example.

> Patrick and Nan came to see me because they were arguing about religion a lot—to the point that they might break up. Patrick was in second-year medicine; Nan in third-year dentistry. They had been living together for a year and a half. Patrick was raised Roman Catholic, but he said that he stopped going to church when he left home to go to college. Nan was raised Baptist but said that she was not religious and hadn't been in a church in years. They did not believe that the faiths in which they were raised were an issue—until Patrick failed his second year of medical school (he was now repeating that year). Like most medical students, Patrick had never failed anything academic in his life. He was deeply embarrassed and guilty about failing, and he took full responsibility for it—that he neglected his studies for sports and extracurricular clubs and groups. He began to attend Sunday Mass. He came away feeling less guilty "for screwing up," and he said that "praying makes me feel more confident that I will do better this year than last year." Nan "freaked" (her words). She said, "Every time Patrick leaves for church, a part of me dies—that I'm losing him. I respect his right to go to church, and I know that it helps him. But I had no idea that he still was Catholic. He was always so negative about the church until now. And he made jokes about the Pope. I'm just really scared. I don't want to make love anymore. And our fights are awful. We get off on tangents and attack each other's families and their beliefs." Patrick agreed: "I find myself defending Catholics and she defends Baptists. It's really nuts. Like a holy war in our tiny apartment. I don't know if either of us really knows what the hell we're fighting about anymore."

Are You Trying to Change Each Other?

Do you want your partner to adopt your ideas, beliefs, or attitudes? How much are you trying to change him or her? How much are you allowing this to simply evolve or unfold over time? Do you feel pressured yourself to attend religious services, observe certain cultural prescriptions, adopt a certain lifestyle, or enjoy particular foodstuffs? If so, are you able to talk about it? Openly and creatively? With resolution, compromises, and insights? Do you feel misunderstood? Defensive? Frightened? Angry? Here is an example of a couple for whom this was a problem.

Harvey was a resident in internal medicine, and Jennifer a final-year medical student. When they came for therapy they had already stopped living together. Jennifer spoke first: "Our relationship was acceptable until Harvey decided he was more Jewish than I thought. Like last Christmas, he agreed to a Christmas tree, so I—we sorta—put one up. Two days later, when I got home from being on call, the tree was taken down—I thought. It was hidden in the closet. Why? Because his father was in town and stopped by to spend a few hours with Harvey. He panicked that his dad might see it, so he hid it. Anyway, that was the beginning of the end. I couldn't ignore any longer that we were different, that we had very different heritages." Harvey cut in: "We have the perfect relationship. Things are not as grim as Jennifer thinks. I'm born Jewish, but I'm not religious. I just think that I need to get used to a Christmas tree. I just need time. I really love Jennifer. It's stupid to give up on something so good as us. I told her that she doesn't need to convert to Judaism, that I'm not trying to change her." Jennifer cut in: "No, not much. What about your thoughts that you want to raise our kids Jewish? That I can continue to go to church—alone—and you will have the kids convert to Judaism and go to synagogue with you? Is that your idea of family? No thanks." Harvey responded: "I just think it's confusing for kids to be raised with two faiths—and then choose when they get older."

I spoke at this point and steered the two of them away from the subject of religion. Their relationship was not as perfect as Harvey believed. In fact, they did not agree on most issues—where they might go for Jennifer's residency if she was not accepted where they lived, their friends, how they managed their finances, their families, how they would get married, and how to relax together. In fact, Harvey dominated their relationship a lot, and Jennifer did not always speak up for herself. She tended to get quiet, withdraw, and pull away sexually. I met with them for several visits, but their paths continued to diverge. They decided to end their relationship.

Here is a couple with ethnic differences but with a different outcome.

Holly and Kamal met as first-year medical students and began dating immediately. They came to see me in third year because they couldn't agree on their wedding plans and living arrangements after marriage. They were fighting a lot, and both got so fed up that they wondered about breaking up, thinking that their differences were insurmountable. They both wanted two weddings—a traditional Indian ceremony in a Hindu temple and a civil ceremony on a beach in Hawaii. However, it was in the details that they were at loggerheads. They were both detailed and perfectionistic people—and neither yielded easily. Their other area of difficulty was where they would live. Kamal felt very strongly that they should live with his aging parents (he had always lived at home, and he wanted Holly to simply move in with him). He stated, "This is my culture. I love my parents. They have lots of room. We would have our own sleeping and studying rooms in the basement and share meals with them upstairs." Holly had not lived at home for eight years, ever since she went off to college. She was quite independent, having traveled alone throughout India between college and medical school, and she lived alone while going to medical school. She said, "Kam, I love your parents too. They are warm and gracious and make me feel like a daughter. I feel very welcome in your family. But my culture is different. We must live on our own. I'm sorry. This is not negotiable."

Here is what happened: Regarding the wedding details "problem," I simply pointed out how I saw each of them and why they were clashing—that is, meticulous, intelligent, creative, exacting, and a little obsessive. I tried to do this in an upbeat way and with a bit of humor. This made them laugh, and I think it eased their tension. They each saw the other as a little "over the top." With this simple explanation, they were able to compromise in a give-and-take way without feeling usurped or bullied by the other. Their talks flowed much more smoothly with this changed attitude.

Their living plans after marriage required much more work. I asked each of them to explain their positions in as much detail as possible and for as long as that took. I requested that they each hear the other out, without interrupting and without trying to punch holes in each other's positions or to change each other's minds. This was difficult for them, and it took several visits and lots of time outside of my office. However, they persevered.

With this exercise, they learned an enormous amount about each other. Not only details about their families and how they grew up but stories—stories that were quite moving and powerful. Lots of feelings came out for each of them—emotions that explained their wishes for independence and autonomy, their need for connection with family, their awe at each other's unique experiences growing up in North America and India, and their conflicts about intimacy with each other. That is, they desired more closeness but were frightened of it at the same time. They came to a point where Kamal was open to living away from home with Holly on their own—and Holly was willing to move into Kamal's family home.

The deciding factor was Kamal's family. His mother and father felt that it was better for the two of them to live on their own. They wanted Kamal not to feel obliged to live with them. They admitted to becoming somewhat acculturated to North America and wanted the house to themselves.

Are Your Families Struggling With Your Relationship?

What do you do if one or both of your families are upset about or don't approve of your relationship? Are you realizing that it's more complicated than simply taking the stance, "That's their problem"? That you are really furious at them? Or deeply hurt? Or embarrassed by their attitude or behavior toward your partner or the two of you? Do you feel caught in the middle between your partner or spouse and your parents?

Here is an example of an interracial marriage, painful at first, that was celebrated later.

Cindy and Charles had been married for six months when they came for marital help because of constant arguing and fighting about Cindy's family. They had lived together for two years before their wedding, which Cindy's parents refused to attend; consequently, they were married in a simple civil ceremony with only a few friends present. Cindy was Asian; Charles Caucasian. Both were graduating in a few months and going away to intern. Charles was bitter and furious at Cindy's parents because they refused to accept him as their son-in-law. He could barely contain his rage, which he also felt guilty about because he knew that Cindy was in the middle. Cindy was quite philosophical; she could empathize with her parents who were immigrants and had never had to face intermarriage with their other children or within their large extended families. She felt that if she continued to talk with her parents and not reject them, over a period of time, they would accept Charles. In fact, she envisioned a "proper wedding" in the future that would be a true celebration of their love and acceptance. This was indeed what happened—two years later.

The marriage of Cindy and Charles is emblematic of how tough a battle it can be for young people in love who are trying to get their families' blessing. Both Cindy and Charles demonstrated phenomenal fortitude and patience as they waited for her parents to come around to acceptance. Some families do not come to this point until the couple has a child. For many, the quest is to explore and uncover spoken and unspoken family rules, prohibitions and taboos, generations of tradition, and deeply held fears of assimilation. Many families are simultaneously mourning and embracing—mourning what once was or a fantasy of what was to be while embracing and trying to condone what is new, foreign, and frightening.

Do Your Classmates Accept Your Relationship?

People in medicine generally tend to be toward the more liberal end of the spectrum of societal prejudice and social stigma. This includes medical students and their professors. However, even the most progressive individuals may individually balk at what to them is different, unexpected, or uncharted. Here are the perceptions of Lloyd and Martha who came to see me about issues around an unplanned pregnancy and resulting conflict in deciding what to do. Lloyd was black and a second-year resident in surgery. Martha was white and a third-year medical student. They were not married but had been coupled for a year and a half.

Lloyd began: "Call me paranoid, but most of my friends who are residents do not approve of my relationship with Martha. I can see it on their faces and in their body language. It's strictly business now when we talk—always about surgery. It didn't use to be that way. We used to talk more about our personal lives, vacations, plans for after residency, and all that. One black woman doctor friend of mine barely speaks to me anymore—like I have really crossed a color line with her, being with a white woman. My attending physicians, I don't really know how they are. At the summer barbecue two weeks ago, people seemed friendly enough to Martha and me, but I noticed that they stared when we were holding hands. I'm black and a minority—I'm very tuned in to that stuff. You really get the sense that people are thinking 'Can't he find a black woman? One of his own?'"

Martha added her perspective: "I laugh—most of the time. Then I just get angry. I really like the classmates that I know. My relationship isn't easy for them, but I think they try. There's some important history here. For over a year, I was in a relationship with a classmate. He was class president, and I was pretty high-profile too because of my sports. We were, for better or worse, nicknamed the 'Ken and Barbie' of our class. When we broke up and soon I was with Lloyd, it was too much for my class, I think. In appearance alone, 'Ken' with his red hair in an 'Archie' cut and his white white skin and Lloyd with his bald head and black skin. I'm not as so-called paranoid as Lloyd, but I do notice that my classmates or Lloyd's resident friends and others do seem to do a double take or stare when they see us together. Funny, I don't see it out in public, like when we're food shopping or at the movies or whatever. I don't know. I guess I expected more of people in medicine."

There are lots of dynamics in intermarriages that present many challenges. I have given a taste in this chapter, but the possibilities are endless. Remember, that we have very little control over whom we fall in love with. We think we do, but that is largely a myth. Intermarriages are rarely deliberately pursued and consciously designed. They happen, and they are largely successful, but as I have illustrated, they pose a dare to societal convention and family values. Hard work, talk and more talk, patience, and opening of hearts ease the journey.

13

I Feel Out of Control

Is It the Relationship or Me?

An unknown number of medical students consult their primary care physician or visit the student health service of their university each year for various symptoms related to the stress of medical training. Of these, a certain percentage go on to have an assessment by a psychiatrist or other mental health professional. What is concerning, however, is that it is estimated that an even larger number of students do not feel well but do not seek help. You may be one of them, or you may know a classmate who carries on despite having trouble sleeping, lots of worries, a bunch of aches and pains, low spirits, failing grades, or heightened use of alcohol or marijuana. It is unfortunate that the stigma of accepting medical illness in oneself, especially mental illness, is so great that many medical students suffer silently.

In this chapter, I want to describe common causes of stress and illnesses in medical students today and to mention some issues and treatments. After you read this chapter, I hope you will be less fearful of reaching out for medical care and will more easily visit your physician when you don't feel well.

Common Psychiatric Diagnoses in Medical Students

The following *DSM-IV* classifications (American Psychiatric Association, 1994) are some of the most common diagnoses made when medical students consult mental health professionals:

- Adjustment disorders, with symptoms of anxiety or depression
- Mood disorders, especially major depressive disorder
- Anxiety disorders—generalized anxiety disorder, panic disorder, various phobias, obsessive compulsive disorder, and posttraumatic stress disorder
- Substance-related disorders, especially related to alcohol and marijuana, as well as to less common prescribed medications such as tranquilizers and sleeping pills or street drugs such as heroin or cocaine
- Eating disorders—anorexia nervosa and bulimia nervosa

These illnesses range all the way from very mild to very severe. Most medical students are not impaired by these conditions, so they are able to do their medical school studies and work safely as long as they are receiving good treatment. However, it is absolutely imperative that you receive treatment if you are suffering from any of these diagnoses, because they will only worsen. Your symptoms will become more severe, you will have trouble concentrating and sleeping, and you will not be able to study properly, use sound medical judgment, and work safely in the medical setting.

A number of other conditions in the *DSM-IV* classification are called V codes. These are conditions with minor psychiatric morbidity, but they may prompt you to visit a mental health professional and receive short-term care. Here are some examples:

- Having trouble communicating with your partner or spouse
- Adjusting to a breakup with your partner or spouse
- Becoming uncomfortable living on your own for the first time, especially if your family lives far away
- Having academic difficulties resulting in poor grades, supplemental exams, or repeating a year of medical school
- Accepting yourself as a gay or lesbian person
- Adopting North American cultural values if you are a fairly recent immigrant from another country

Do You Have a Problem With Alcohol?

One of the cardinal features of alcohol dependence or abuse is denial in the individual. In other words, you may not or will not be able to see it in yourself. This is not uncommon in medical students who very quickly are able to rationalize their use of alcohol. The most common rationalization is that they are no different from their classmates or other young people their age whom they describe as drinking as much as they do or even more. One way that you can be helped with your denial is if people are more concerned about your drinking than you are. This is also classic. And if one of these individuals is your partner or spouse, you must pay attention to his or her concerns—even if he or she is a teetotaler.

It is unusual for medical students to be diagnosed with substance misuse or dependence. However, addiction medicine research reveals that many physicians who have been diagnosed with and are being treated for alcohol or other drugs of dependence give a history that they began to use excessively during medical school or even earlier during their adolescence. They did not recognize it as a problem then, and sometimes no one else did either. If you are an older medical student, you may have the maturity and insight to realize that you were beginning to develop a problem with alcohol or drugs earlier and have dealt with that accordingly. Or you may already be very active in a recovery program.

Teaching about alcoholism and other drugs of dependence has improved substantially in North American medical schools over the past two decades. This is done both didactically and clinically, so your knowledge base about this subject should be quite sound. Be open to looking inward at your own personal use of alcohol and other drugs, your partner's or spouse's, and your family's use of chemicals. It is well-known that a significant percentage of today's medical students have family members who suffer from alcoholism or other forms of drug abuse or dependence, and for genetic reasons alone, many of you will be at risk. You must treat alcohol and other drugs with caution and with respect. Excessive use of alcohol and other drugs is one of the most common causes of relationship discord and relationship breakdown in our society. Medical students are no exception. Here is an example.

Paul, a fourth-year medical student, came to see me after being charged with impaired driving and having his driver's license suspended. His wife Clair had been trying unsuccessfully to get him to seek treatment for alcoholism for at least two years. He often drank too much, especially on weekends. During these times, he was boisterous, touchy, and sarcastic. Not only with Clair but with her friends as well. He had "blackouts" during these episodes, but because he never struck Clair and never drank when on call, he considered his drinking "no different from that of any other medical student." His father, one brother, two paternal uncles, and two maternal aunts were severely alcoholic. He dismissed this as "unimportant."

Like Paul and Clair above, most medical students in marriages in which one or both have a problem with alcohol or drugs have marital difficulties as a consequence. In fact, many students, unfortunately, will not face the problem until their spouses are so worn out, furious, and demoralized that they leave the relationship, or threaten to, unless something is done. In my practice, I occasionally see medical student couples who have come with what appears to be a straightforward problem with communication. However, I quickly realize and point out to them that it is impossible to have good communication if and when one of them has had more than a social drink or a fair amount of marijuana.

The stigma associated with having an alcohol or other drug problem when you are a medical student reinforces the denial. However, these days, many medical schools have peer support programs for students who have a substance dependence problem, which can be very helpful and also go a long way toward reducing the shame and guilt associated with abuse of drugs. These programs usually also have links with community recovery programs for physicians, such as Alcoholics Anonymous, Narcotics Anonymous, Caduceus groups, Adult Children of Alcoholics groups, and so on. It is very important to remember that most medical students and residents who seek treatment for chemical dependency do very well in terms of becoming and remaining "clean and sober."

Drinking too much or using too many drugs is rarely due to a primary marital problem. You may be drinking more or using more drugs in an attempt to cope with an unhappy or miserable relationship, but you were probably vulnerable before using drugs to excess. What is much more common is that drugs and alcohol cause relationship heartache.

Are You Depressed?

You should see your doctor if you develop four or more of the following symptoms that last more than two weeks:

- Change of appetite—weight loss or weight gain
- Change in sleep
- •Loss of interest and pleasure in your usual activities
- Loss of energy or you feel tired easily

- Feelings of worthlessness
- Feelings of hopelessness
- Inability to concentrate, indecisiveness
- Thoughts of death and suicide
- Melancholia—deep sadness, grief feelings
- Irrational thinking, obsessive ruminations
- Physical symptoms (stomach trouble, headaches, backaches)

Your primary care physician will do a complete assessment, which may include a visit with your spouse or partner, and he or she will make a diagnosis and suggest treatment. Treatment often includes medication—an antidepressant—and supportive psychotherapy. Depending on the stressors and other factors that may be contributing to your depression, your primary care physician may recommend referral to a psychiatrist or other mental health professional for other types of psychotherapy, such as interpersonal, cognitive-behavioral, marital, family, or group therapy.

If you or your spouse or partner are suffering from a mood disorder, you are more prone to marital distress, conflict, and marital breakdown than someone who does not have this type of illness. It is therefore extremely important that you or your loved one have an assessment and receive proper treatment. Relationships are already a major challenge in our society. Why not get help if you have a mood disorder that aggravates the problem?

We also know that in a certain percentage of couples, both partners have psychiatric disorder. For instance, one of you may suffer from a mood disorder and your partner has a panic disorder, an eating disorder, or a mood disorder, too. So life together can feel quite precarious. It is difficult to be an involved husband or wife when you don't feel well, when you're depressed, when you're intoxicated with alcohol, when you've got a social phobia, or when you have obsessive-compulsive disorder and have to check all of the burners on the stove, all of the light switches in the house, or all of the water faucets in your apartment six times before you can leave for medical school classes in the morning.

Sometimes it is the other way around; an unhappy relationship or a relationship that is full of conflict can affect your mental health. In other words, marital strain can make you sick. Usually, this is very obvious. For example, you know that you are feeling depressed because you and your partner are fighting constantly; you're having trouble sleeping because your husband is late again and you suspect he might be having an affair; you are having panic attacks because you and your wife have just separated; your self-esteem is the pits because you strongly.suspect that your girlfriend is lesbian; you started to drink more because your wife had a therapeutic abortion that you did not agree with.

Sometimes, however, you may not be able to see that you have a problem or problems in your relationship. You may be somebody who tends to blame himself or herself for everything, and you cannot see that your partner is partly responsible and that the two of you really do have a relationship problem. In other words, it takes a close friend, a family member, or a professional to help you understand that your depressed mood, your agoraphobia, or your headaches are because your husband is never home before midnight, that he does not help out with the children, that he subtly puts you down, and that he does not respect you as an equal in the relationship.

What About Eating Disorders?

Unfortunately, eating disorders are not uncommon in women medical students. They also occasionally occur in male medical students. Although eating disorders range from mild to very severe, they always have an impact on one's significant relationship. It is very hard for the partner or spouse of someone with an eating disorder not to be worried. It is also not uncommon for there to be fights over food and a lot of worry that your wife may starve herself to death or become metabolically ill from the repeated overeating, vomiting, or purging associated with bulimia. And there's the terror that she may kill herself.

It is normal then to be anxious or frustrated if your wife has an eating disorder. It may be very hard for you to ignore her eating problems. If she is in no immediate danger, though, you will have to step back and let her work with her doctor and nutritionist with regard to her weight. You probably know that unless you let go, your vigilance or interfering introduces too much control into your relationship. Furthermore, it casts you into the role of a parent, and this role is never healthy in marriage. Your wife's therapists are probably doing their best to let her function as independently as possible and take back control of her own life. Although it may appear to you that this is very self-destructive, this is a process that takes time. If, on the other hand, your wife is seriously deteriorating and is very ill and totally unable to appreciate how life threatening her behavior is, you will have to intervene and get in touch with her physician. Your wife's physician should understand that you are not overreacting or being overcontrolling but that you are merely being human. It is very important that you and your wife's physician or physicians have a mutually respectful relationship.

It will help you to look inward to see whether or not you might be "co-dependent." No one likes this label. However, you may be inadvertently reinforcing your wife's problem by doing things that make it worse: telling her that she's too fat or too thin; reprimanding her for eating this or that; controlling her in another area of your marriage, which may be in part aggravating her eating problem; needing her to be sick so that you can feel strong, fulfilling a need that you have to be the caretaker. You may find it helpful to read one of the many books that are available on codependency. If you have alcoholism or drug dependence in your family, you may very well be codependent.

You may also benefit from therapy yourself. It is extremely difficult living with someone with an eating disorder. Are there support groups available in your community for family members of individuals with an eating disorder? It is also possible that you and your wife could benefit from marital therapy. There may be other problems that need addressing that could indirectly be related to your wife's eating disorder. You may also benefit from the guidance of a couples therapist to approach issues that are difficult for you and your wife to talk about. Here are some other issues the two of you could discuss in marital therapy:

- The lying and deception that goes on with your wife's eating disorder
- The mistrust that you have for your wife
- The sense you have of being manipulated
- Whether you have a concern or fear that your wife may kill herself
- Your wife's perception of you as controlling
- Your wife's fear that you will abandon her
- You wife's wish to be more aware of her feelings
- Your wife's wish to be more mature and responsible for her actions
- Your sadness about how the eating disorder has affected your marriage or has dominated your partnership
- For both of you, a sense of exhaustion and demoralization because of the chronicity of your wife's illness
- For both of you, mourning for the good times that you used to have together
- Concern that your intimacy has been destroyed
- Concern about your sexual relationship
- Concern that your marriage is coming to an end

Reference

American Psychiatric Association. (1994). *Diagnostic and statistical manual of mental disorders* (4th ed.). Washington, DC: Author.

14 Looking Ahead to Residency

If you have started your last two years of medical school, you are probably beginning to think about residency—what field you might pursue and where you might apply to do your training. These are central and critical life decisions, and if you are in a relationship, you will be doing lots of talking with your spouse or partner. He or she may have lots of thoughts and feelings about what residency you are interested in, how much you seem to like or love that branch of medicine, how time intensive it is, whether or not you need to move from where you are living now to another city, and so forth. Lots of relationship variables will shape your decision and your talks with each other. What follows is a list of questions:

- How long have you been a couple, and what is the state of your relationship? How committed are you to each other?

- If you are married or similarly committed, is it a given that your decision about your residency will be made only after lots of discussion with each other?

- Despite being married or similarly committed, is it possible that you might end your relationship through the process of deciding on a residency? In other words, is your relationship in trouble or perhaps "over" without either of you really acknowledging it, and separating at graduation is perhaps a socially acceptable way of calling it quits?

- How do you communicate with each other about such important matters? Is deciding on your residency essentially a "we" decision or a "me" decision, with your partner or spouse simply following without much input?

- How "portable" is your partner or spouse if you have to move to a program in another city? If he or she absolutely cannot move because of work or family commitments, that is obviously a very important matter that restricts your options and application process.

- If you are classmates, how much are you taking each other into consideration in terms of where you apply and to what programs you apply? Should you have concerns if you are both interested in residencies with very long hours and frequent on-call responsibilities such as surgery or surgical subspecialties? Do you have fears that your relationship can sustain that degree of professional commitment and still survive?

These few questions touch on some of the many issues that characterize medical student relationships at this point in training. Each year in my practice, I see a number of medical student couples who are struggling with and negotiating these or similar dynamics. Indeed, the professional life stage of approaching the end of medical school and contemplating or beginning residency can be very stressful, despite the relief and excitement of graduating. The intimate relationships of many medical students are put to the test. Some don't make it, and that's OK; some don't make it, and that's not OK; and some do make it, and that's very OK because there is growth and deepening intimacy through the process.

Should Being Married Influence My Choice of Residency?

In absolute terms, no. You have to follow your heart, your gut, your soul, what makes you feel good, what branch of medicine stimulates you—since you want or hope to enjoy your work for your whole medical career. If you are not fulfilled professionally and do not love what you do (most of the time), you are not going to be such a great partner in a relationship, and vice versa, if you are not happy at home, it is hard to really enjoy your residency. Healthy relationships provide sustenance and support during the long years of training.

When contemplating your residency, ask yourself all or some of these questions:

- How much time will this program give me to have a life outside of medicine?
- How "relationship-friendly" is this particular program?
- How much importance do I attach to my intimate relationship? Am I prepared to fight for balance in this branch of medicine to give my relationship the time and energy that all relationships require?

- Have I accepted any health limitations that I have or that my spouse has—for example, diabetes, multiple sclerosis, cancer, mood disorder, alcoholism, and so forth? Might the specifics of certain branches of medicine put me (or him or her) at risk for relapse or exacerbation of symptoms?

- My heart is set on being a cardiologist (or a urologist, an ophthalmologist, a radiologist, an anesthesiologist, etc.). How do I know if I am just paying lip service to my relationship and simply expecting my spouse or partner to be supportive, strong, uncomplaining, and patient?

- How much does my partner or spouse fully understand the demands of this program? Has he or she truly researched it? Is he or she able to make an informed decision, or is he or she being naive and urging me "to go for it" without a lot of thought?

- (If you have children or contemplate having children during residency) How family-friendly is this program? Is there a parental leave policy? What is their attitude toward pregnant residents and "expectant" fathers? Can I stay home, without guilt, if my son or daughter is sick?

- Have I talked to any current residents in this branch of medicine about lifestyle matters, in particular how much time they get to spend with their partners or spouses?

- What kind of relationship breakdown rate occurs in this program? Higher than average? What is the divorce rate of physicians in this branch of medicine? Are the demands of this branch of medicine felt to play a role in relationship morbidity?

There are no easy answers to these questions, but you need to ask them. You need to ask them of yourself, your partner, and others in your considered field of study. Specialty programs still have a long way to go in terms of honoring the personal lives of their trainees. With few exceptions, they are still largely designed for the unattached person, the physician who is able and prepared to work and study an enormous number of hours per week for at least four years to become a first-rate clinician. Our programs are out of step with the realities of today. How many applicants are unattached and/or still will be when they complete their training? It is shameful that so many relationships do not survive residency training. It is even more shameful that we are so loath to acknowledge it, to address it, and to implement preventative measures.

Ted had wanted to be a surgeon since he was in high school. His mother died of breast cancer when he was 15 years old, and losing her had a profound effect on him. Mary, the daughter of a surgeon and a college professor, was a music teacher in a high school. Ted and Mary had been married for a year when they came to see me. They had only one complaint—their arguing and disagreements over Ted's plan to apply for a residency in surgery. Mary's stance was that Ted was naive, that he had no idea of the lifestyle choice he was making, that he would have to sacrifice a lot of his personal interests for his career, and that he would not be able to be the involved husband and father that he envisioned. Mary admitted that she was far from objective. Her father was a "workaholic" surgeon ("I don't know him, I grew up fatherless, he drinks too much, he's arrogant and selfish, I think he cheats on my mother"). She said, "And I don't want to become like my mother—lonely, bitter, bitchy, and depressed." I asked Ted to speak to some of the residents in surgery at his medical school and to some of his attending physicians. What they had to say was not as grim as Mary's perspective, but they did tell him that life was not rosy, that they all worked very hard, that they had little time for sports, and that there were lots of divorced and remarried residents and surgeons attached to the program. Ted applied to surgery and was matched at a program in another city. In the end, Mary was happy for him and they moved. I never saw them again. However, I did receive a letter from them two years later. They had separated but had reconciled. Ted had dropped out of the program after a year and started a residency in pathology. He was still adjusting to this "because I really miss surgery—but not the drudgery," and Mary was pregnant with their first child. They were happy and getting along well.

*   *   *

Jim and Holly were in the same class and had been living together for over a year when they came to see me. Their initial plans to both apply for psychiatry residency seemed great until Jim began to demur. He wasn't sure if they should attempt to match together at the same program or even if he wanted to do psychiatry. My sessions with the two of them were focused on helping Jim to clarify what he really wanted—because his ups and downs and "mind games" were very hard on Holly. She wasn't sleeping, was getting panic attacks, and couldn't concentrate on her clinical work and studying. After a few visits, it became increasingly clear that Jim wanted out of the relationship, that he wasn't as certain of their future together as he had felt, that he wasn't ready to "settle down," and that he was looking at residency as "an adventure—the next phase of my life—without the responsibility of a relationship." As he became more direct with Holly, she felt a lot better—sad and angry but not so anxious and preoccupied. She had lots of support in their class (and from her family). She asked Jim to move out, and he was OK with that. They applied to programs in psychiatry in different cities. Our paths have crossed at medical meetings, and they each seem to be doing well.

* * *

Kate had been accepted into an OB-GYN residency when she and her husband Matthew came to see me. Their challenge was facing a commuter marriage. Kate was not matched locally, and she would be living a one-hour flight away. Matthew had his own business, and he argued that he could not move. Kate was very unhappy about this and did not accept his rationale at all. She took his resistance very personally and had many insecurities and accusations—that he didn't really love her, that he was not really committed to the marriage, that he had duped her, that he was probably going to date other women, and so on. She was very angry and very scared. Matthew was dumbfounded by her barrage of attacks, and because he wasn't very verbal or very articulate, his attempts to explain himself were confusing and not at all reassuring to Kate. This formed much of our therapy. I helped Matthew (by paraphrasing what I thought he was trying to say) to assert himself and to speak more directly and more intimately to Kate. I simultaneously tried to help Kate tone down her attacks on Matthew's character by asking her to speak more about her feelings of fear, infidelity, loneliness, abandonment, and guilt. It was also helpful for Kate to recognize that much of what she was experiencing was a reliving of a very painful state when her father left the family when she was 14 years old (interestingly, her father was also an OB-GYN, and he left Kate's mother and began living with one of his residents!). Matthew's stance was rooted in financial worry and insecurity—he grew up in a very conservative, struggling, and hard-working family. His father worked at the same company for 45 years! For Matthew to sell his business and move to the city of Kate's training was very frightening—almost overwhelming. But that is what he did—during

Kate's second year of residency—after they successfully commuted for about 18 months, seeing each other about every three to four weeks.

Suggestions

- Talk to your spouse or partner as early as possible when you begin thinking about residency.
- Remember that your initial talk or talks, and the conclusions you reach, must be seen as just that—the beginning of a process. You each have every right to change your mind as your discussions unfold and evolve.
- If your relationship is solid and you are both committed to each other, your deliberations will be easier. It is a given that you are equally concerned about and sensitive to the wishes of each other and that your discussions will have a give-and-take form.
- If your relationship is "young," the process of exploring residency options and sites (both on your own and with each other) will have a huge impact on whether your relationship "makes" it or not. You may conclude that it is impossible to do both and you go your separate ways. You may find that your love for each other deepens with looking ahead to residency, and you may marry each other. Or you may find that you go off to your residency in an ambiguous state of uncertainty— together or alone—with the thought of "time will tell."
- If your relationship is wobbly (a.k.a. in trouble, unhappy, rancorous, tension filled, conflict ridden, bogged down, etc.), you may use residency as an opportunity to get out of it and if married, to divorce. This could be face-saving for both of you. And if your health and well-being has been affected by your relationship, separating will be a wise decision. You will still need to mourn, but at least you will be starting your residency afresh.

15

Surely We Can Fix This Ourselves

I'm a Medical Student!

In this chapter, I want to address some of the more common reactions to stress in a relationship. You have recognized that you and your partner or spouse are having a problem, but the problem does not seem to be going away, or if it does, it returns again and again. Or a new problem arises that upsets your stability as a couple.

The Question of Marital Therapy

The notion of seeking some professional help has arisen. Here's a not uncommon situation:

She says: Let's go see someone about our relationship. We're both miserable.

He says: We don't need marital counseling. We can figure this out ourselves.

She says: That's what we have been trying for a long time. It's not working.

He says: That's because you never listen to me. I keep telling you that you're too emotional. You need to calm down.

She says: Yes—and become the constipated logician that you are. Stop trying to control me!

He says: Stop accusing me of trying to control you. I'm just asking you to use your brain. How can someone as smart as you be so stupid?

She says: And how can someone as stupid as you be so arrogant!?

He says: You know, you can be a real bitch sometimes, can't you?

She says: See why we need counseling? We can't even talk about counsel-
            ing without fighting.

The above dialogue isn't uncommon in male-female relationships that are in trouble. The woman decides that things are not working and that attempts to settle things on their own are not working. She is open to seeing a therapist together, but the man's initial reaction is as above. Many men, and some women, have the mistaken belief that intelligence and reason are all that's necessary to make communication flow in an intimate relationship. These two qualities help, but they can also hinder. Sometimes individuals who are highly intelligent, articulate, and logical, people with Ph.D.s in communication theory and who are intimately involved with each other can't even talk about the weather without fighting. In the example above, the man is really saying (but not saying), "I'm afraid of therapy—talking about such personal stuff with a complete stranger." Or "I'm embarrassed. I'm a medical student, for God's sake. A therapist is going to think that we're really stupid that we can't talk about the simplest things without wanting to strangle each other."

I'm Too Busy to Go for Help.
Exams Are Coming.

This is a common cop-out in medical student relationships. In other words, the pressures, demands, responsibilities, and time constraints of medical school become a convenient excuse for all kinds of things—in this case, working on one's intimate relationship. No wonder that many partners and spouses of medical students question where they are on that person's list of priorities. Am I important to you or not? Do you care enough about me or us to go with me for help or not? What's more important—yourself and your education or us?

Herein lies a paradox. Making the time for couples therapy will free up time for studying. In other words, improving your relationship with each other translates into more efficient communication and less time wasted worrying, crying, arguing, or withdrawing angrily—not to mention that feeling happier and more confident about one's relationship makes work and study easier, maybe even enjoyable.

Another cop-out is refusing to go for help and sending your partner for help because he or she is or seems more upset. If the problem is the two of you, how can only one of you going for help work? And yet this is very common. Many primary care physicians and mental health professionals are referred individuals each year whose source of symptoms is their relationship—and their partner refuses to attend. My advice to you? GO WITH YOUR PARTNER! Even if you think that it's all your partner's problem (which is never so but is a common belief nonetheless), you will gain something from the experience.

I Promise to
Give Up Marijuana—Today!

This is another form of resistance to couples therapy. That is, one of you promises to change something that really bothers the other or something that has been an irritant in your lives together. As noble as the intention is, it rarely works—for two reasons. First, usually it is not so easy to suddenly stop doing something. Second, giving something up is usually only part of the problem. Either there are underlying or associated issues that need addressing, or the partner also has liabilities that need examining. Here are some quotations from medical student couples about behaviors that are not so easy to simply stop doing without professional help:

- I know you're furious, and you're right. I always keep you waiting. Well, never again. I will never be late again.

- I know you think I can't stop drinking. I don't agree, but because it bugs you so much I'm going to stop drinking today. I'll show you that I can take it or leave it.

- My eating disorder hasn't come back. I don't really need to make myself vomit after meals. I can stop it if it bugs you so much.

- I promise. I'm so sorry, please forgive me. I feel so guilty. Don't worry. I will never hit you again—never.

- That's it. I really get it now after what happened last night at the party. I promise that I'll keep my hands off other women. I've grown up. I don't need to prove anything anymore.

- Mark my words, I promise to never call you a _____ again, no matter how angry I am.

- We don't need to see anyone about our sexual relationship. I won't make you wait so long anymore for sex. Just let me know and we'll do it.

My advice to you: Try to see the possible underlying reasons for these issues and discuss them. You might be able to help each other simultaneously work on things. Give yourselves a few weeks. If there is no change, get some help.

Let's Just Break Up

One more type of resistance to formal help is the thought of "pulling the plug." It comes from being exhausted, demoralized, and feeling hopeless. There is a need for relief from the constant conflict, tension, sadness, and emptiness. Breaking up offers that. Or does it? In some cases, no—because you may be no happier on your own. It is best to get an opinion from an expert in couples or family therapy. You may have a viable relationship and don't know it. A professional should be able to help you with that question. And if your relationship is truly over, he or she should be able to determine that.

If you are not married or cohabiting, you may be tempted to just call it quits, thinking that if you need professional help, you should not even be together, that there is something fundamentally wrong with your relationship. This is not always true. It is really a matter of degree. Many couples can be helped with "premarital counseling." In fact, it is wise to address some of these very basic issues before a further commitment rather than sweep them away only for them to resurface later, after one or two children. And if you have been married before (or have experienced the breakup of a serious and committed relationship akin to marriage), you can benefit greatly from couples therapy in your current relationship. Why? Because you really want this relationship to work; you don't want to relive the heartache of another breakup.

16 Is There Any Decent Help Out There?

The answer, of course, is yes. But cynicism is rampant in our society about the value of professional help and its practitioners. And medical students and their partners are not immune to cynicism themselves. Here are some of the most common reasons why embracing professional help is so hard:

• One or each of you is very private, and talking with someone about something as personal as your relationship is a very private matter. You will need a sense that whomever you see is respectful of you and this basic tenet. Remember that therapy can proceed only in a safe, private, confidential context.

• You are embarrassed or ashamed of something. This may be simple embarrassment that your relationship is strained and you can't seem to fix it on your own. Or you may feel embarrassed about a problem that you have or that your partner has that is one of the factors in your discord or unhappiness with each other. Here are some examples: You have premature ejaculation. You have an eating disorder. You are having an affair. You are a crossdresser. You are bisexual. You have genital herpes. You were sexually abused as a child. You have had a therapeutic abortion. Your mother was a prostitute. Your father has a criminal record. You were on social assistance in the past. The list is endless.

• You may tend to be self-reliant. You don't turn to others easily for assistance. Your background and style has been to figure things out for yourself, and that has served you well so far in life. This may be the first time in your life that, despite all of your efforts to resolve things with your partner, it isn't working.

• You may have had a negative experience with therapy. Or someone in your family did. If you had a falling out with a previous therapist or if you felt "picked on" or found that therapy didn't seem to help or seemed to make things worse, you may be reluctant to enter that world again with your spouse or partner. Understandably, you would need to research whom you might go to see, and I would advise you to speak about your reservations in your first visit with that individual.

• You are proud and perfectionistic. Going for professional help makes you feel flawed or "less than." As a medical student, and future physician, you feel you should not have any problems—and if you do, you must keep them under wraps.

• Stigma is getting to you. Seeing a cardiologist is OK, but seeing a psychiatrist or other mental health professional is not. Perhaps you struggle with internalized feelings of stigma—that people who see psychiatrists are losers, weak, or crazy. And they don't make very good doctors.

• You don't respect mental health professionals. You view practitioners through stereotypic eyes; that is, social workers are all a bunch of do-gooders, psychologists are wanna-be doctors, and psychiatrists are not real physicians.

Going with your spouse or partner for help may be one of the most important things that you can do for your relationship. It is very helpful to meet with someone who is outside your relationship, someone who can objectively interpret what's going on. And yes, it takes guts and maturity to reach out for assistance—and trust in the process, that this individual has both of your best interests at heart.

Where Can We Get Help?

There are lots of variables here, and the options open to you will depend on your medical school, health insurance, and personal resources.

• *Office of student advocacy.* In most medical schools, the office of student affairs is headed by one of the associate deans. Medical schools vary in the range and breadth of counseling services available to students who are having personal difficulties. Much of this will be covered at orientation to medical school, and whom to call and so on will be recorded in your written materials.

Class presidents and peer counselors in medical school can usually answer questions about how or where to get help. REMEMBER: Any counseling or therapy that you and your spouse or partner might receive is completely confidential. Individuals who treat you, even if they have an academic appointment, have no connection with your academic record whatsoever. This would constitute a conflict of interest and is unethical.

• *Student health service.* All universities have health services for students. Once again, confidentiality applies as above. This service is usually staffed by a team of health professionals: primary care physicians and nurses, medical specialists (including psychiatrists subspecialized in student health), and other mental health professionals (e.g., psychologists, social workers, family counselors, clergy, and so forth). If one of you were to visit a primary care physician, he or she would assess your situation and determine what, if any, medical investigation and treatment is necessary and then suggest other services. Here is an example:

Daphne, a second-year medical student, went to see her physician at the student health office because she was losing weight, had developed a tremor, was feeling very nervous and sweaty in class, and had become claustrophobic on elevators. She also wasn't sleeping very well and startled easily. Her physician, after taking a complete medical history and examining her, told her that she wanted to do some tests to rule out hyperthyroidism. She was also wondering about a psychiatric illness: anxiety disorder or perhaps depression. Daphne began crying. She too was worried about her mental health. Her husband, a law clerk, was working very hard, was late every night, and had stopped wanting to make love. She strongly suspected that he was having an affair. When he denied it but nothing changed, Daphne wondered if she was "losing it." Her physician referred her to a psychiatrist on staff who interviewed Daphne's husband for collaborative information: He disclosed that he indeed was involved with a woman at work and was now prepared to tell Daphne about that. The psychiatrist referred the two of them to a psychologist on staff for marital therapy.

• *Psychiatrists.* You may decide that you wish to see a psychiatrist about your relationship. You should determine ahead of time whether the person you wish to see or to whom you are referred does indeed do couples therapy or whether that is covered under your health insurance. If you have both a clinical depression and a relationship problem, your psychiatrist will want to treat your depression first (or perhaps simultaneously). This probably will mean taking an antidepressant. Even if your depression is partly or largely due to relationship strain, listen carefully to your psychiatrist's advice about medication. Why? Because it is really tough, if not impossible, to work at couples therapy if you have lots of symptoms of depression: You aren't sleeping properly, you are tired a lot, you have trouble concentrating, you are more sensitive than usual, you feel extremely vulnerable and frightened, and so forth. Taking medication does not remove your motivation for or ability to engage in therapy. That is a myth!

• *Nonmedical therapists.* This includes psychologists, social workers, marital and family counselors, and the clergy. These individuals make up the bulk of professionals who do couples therapy. Most have a master's degree or a doctorate. Be certain to ask your therapist about his or her credentials, training, and membership in professional associations and societies.

Conclusion

Try to take a proactive and positive approach to couples therapy. Look at your therapist as a consultant, someone you have hired to help the two of you work on your relationship—not as someone with all the answers, not as someone who knows what's best for the two of you, not as someone who is going to tell you what to do. Each of you should feel heard and respected by your therapist. If you feel that he or she is not being objective, fair, or neutral, speak up! If you feel singled out, picked on, or judged, say so! If you feel that therapy isn't helping or that things are worse (remembering though that sometimes things may get worse before they get better), discuss this with your therapist. And finally, remember that the goal of couples therapy is for each of you to feel clearer about yourself and each other whatever form this may take. Couples therapy is not about preserving relationships at all costs. If your relationship is a viable one with potential for growth, mutual respect, and enduring love, couples therapy will improve your communication with each other, expedite change, and reinforce your commitment. If your relationship is not healthy or not good for BOTH of you, couples therapy will help to increase your realization and acceptance of that. And it should assist you in going your separate ways with dignity and less pain.

Suggested Readings

Beck, A. (1988). *Love is never enough: How couples can overcome misunderstandings, resolve conflicts, and solve relationship problems through cognitive therapy.* New York: Harper & Row.

Gabbard, G. O., & Menninger, R. W. (1988). *Medical marriages.* Washington, DC: American Psychiatric Press.

Myers, M. F. (1994). *Doctors' marriages: A look at the problems and their solutions* (2nd ed.). New York: Plenum.

Myers, M. F. (1998). *How's your marriage? A book for men and women.* Washington, DC: American Psychiatric Press.

Peterkin, A. D. (1998). *Staying human during residency training* (2nd ed.). Toronto, Ontario: University of Toronto Press.

Sotile, W. M., & Sotile, M. O. (2000). *The medical marriage.* (2nd ed.). Chicago: American Medical Association.

Tannen, D. (1990). *You just don't understand: Women and men in conversation.* New York: William Morrow.

Index

About the Author

Michael F. Myers, M.D., is Director of the Marital Therapy Clinic at St. Paul's Hospital in Vancouver, British Columbia, Canada, and Clinical Professor in the Department of Psychiatry at the University of British Columbia. Dr. Myers has written three previous books, *Doctors' Marriages: A Look at the Problems and Their Solutions; Men and Divorce;* and *How's Your Marriage? A Book for Men and Women* and has coedited with Larry Goldman, M.D., and Leah Dickstein, M.D., *The Handbook of Physician Health.* He has also written several scientific publications and book chapters and produced educational videotapes on marriage, divorce, medical student and physician stress, abuse of residents, sexual assault of women and men, AIDS, the stigma of psychiatric illness, boundary issues in the physician-patient relationship, gender issues in health care and delivery, and physician suicide and its impact on loved ones. Active in many medical associations, Dr. Myers currently serves on the Board of Trustees of the American Psychiatric Association and is President-Elect of the Canadian Psychiatric Association.

Printed in the United States
By Bookmasters